Sinusitis

Dr Paul Carson is a member of the British Society for Allergy & Clinical Immunology and the European Academy of Allergology and Clinical Im ology. He is a board member of the Irish Lung Foundation and an   ry member of the Severe Asthma Advisory Group in Ireland. He has   five other self-help books for adults and children on allergy-related   <www.allergy-ireland.ie>

Overcoming Common Problems Series

Selected titles

A full list of titles is available from Sheldon Press,
36 Causton Street, London SW1P 4ST and on our website at
www.sheldonpress.co.uk

Overcoming Common Problems Series

Overcoming Common Problems Series

Overcoming Common Problems

Sinusitis
Steps to healing

DR PAUL CARSON

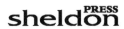
sheldon **PRESS**

First published in Great Britain in 2009
Sheldon Press
36 Causton Street
London SW1P 4ST

The author and publisher have made every effort to ensure that the
external website and email addresses included in this book are correct and
up to date at the time of going to press. The author and publisher are not
responsible for the content, quality or continuing accessibility of the sites.

British Library Cataloguing-in-Publication Data
A catalogue record for this book is available from the British Library

ISBN 978–1–84709–087–4

1 3 5 7 9 10 8 6 4 2

Typeset by Fakenham Photosetting Ltd, Fakenham, Norfolk
Printed in Great Britain by Ashford Colour Press

Produced on paper from sustainable forests

To Jean

Note: This is not a medical book and is not intended to replace advice from your doctor. Do consult your doctor if you are experiencing symptoms with which you feel you need help.

Contents

Introduction

You're feeling miserable and it's not for the first time this year. Your nose is bunged up; you have a headache and a completely different sort of pain running along the top of your teeth. Your sense of smell is poor and most foods taste like cardboard. You're exhausted and can't sleep properly from snorting and snoring and clearing your throat. Your partner has fled to the silence of the spare bedroom. So you go to the doctor.

'I think I've got another sinus –'

And he has a prescription for an antibiotic written almost before you can add '– infection.'

You look at the scribble and recognize it's the same antibiotic prescribed the last time. And the time before that. It didn't work then and you're not convinced it will work this time.

'Look doctor, I don't want to be a moan but this is the third time I've had to visit you this year with sinusitis.' You flap the prescription in the air. 'Is there anything else I can do?'

'Well, you could try a decongestant, or maybe inhale some eucalyptus oil vapour. Have you considered acupuncture?' But he doesn't sound convincing, the advice more like a spiel used often before.

By now your nose is dripping, your head is pounding and you realize you've forgotten to bring tissues. You resist the temptation to use the sleeve of your blouse. You take a big sniff and say, 'Maybe I should see a specialist?' You're pushing to be taken seriously.

'You mean an ear, nose and throat surgeon?'

'Ear, nose and throat *surgeon*?' 'Well, maybe ... perhaps.' Surgery? Suddenly this doesn't seem like a good idea after all.

'Yes, surgery might be indicated,' says the doctor, trying to be helpful. 'It could indeed sort you out.' He starts preparing a referral to the local ear, nose and throat (ENT) department. But this doesn't cheer you up because you've heard horror stories about sinus surgery and you want to get better, not be made worse. So you force a brave smile and politely decline. 'Actually no, I don't much fancy having my facial bones drilled.'

'Me neither,' he says. He's on his feet and opening the door. The consultation is over.

An hour later you're standing in the pharmacy, checking the rows of non-prescription remedies and wondering which one might just work this time. And you're quietly screaming *help*.

And I've heard you. You're not alone.

Sinus problems are real, debilitating, painful and often stubborn to clear. But there is a treatment plan for everybody, including you. Or rather, especially you, now that you've reached this line. You are fed up. And you're fed up feeling fed up and unwell.

But there have been significant advances in our under-standing of the condition. Using special X-rays and flexible fibre optics we now realize just how much swelling, obstruction and fluid blistering there is in aggressive sinusitis. And we also have the knowledge to correct this.

This book will take you through all the remedies for sinusitis, conventional and unorthodox, and gently tease you along the correct path to good health. I will touch on surgery for certain stub-born sinus conditions. However, the good news is that nowadays surgery is less important than appropriate medical remedies.

You might be tempted to jump straight to the chapter on treatments. Please don't. Take time to read how your sinuses work and what happens when they stop working (and why). Being informed allows you to better understand the therapies available.

I've focused only on common problems, for this is not a text-book. There are other rare and unusual conditions that produce sinus-type symptoms. The doctor who treats you must decide if your symptoms suggest more detailed investigation than explained on these pages.

I've been dealing with nose and sinus problems in children and adults for over 25 years. Let me offer my experience to help you learn to love your sinuses once again.

Dr Paul Carson
Dublin, Ireland

1

How sinusitis happens and what other medical conditions it can trigger

'I think I have a sinus problem.'

You may well have, but it's probably not the only difficulty. *Almost all sinus problems begin inside the nose.* If you read that sentence again and again throughout this book it's only because I do want to labour the point. *Almost all sinus problems begin inside the nose.*

So let's start with some basic understanding of your sinuses, where they're located, how they function and their link to the nose.

The sinuses are cave-like structures inside the bony skull. They cluster around the nose (as shown in Figures 1.1 to 1.4) and connect directly with the inside lining of the nose via small tubes. These tubes must stay clear to allow the sinuses to 'breathe' and drain. If they become obstructed then problems occur. The mucous membrane in the nose and sinuses is our personal air conditioner, cleaning and filtering and humidifying inhaled air before it enters the lungs. It is extremely delicate and easily damaged.

Figure 1.1 is a diagram of where the sinuses are located.

The sinuses are lined with much the same material as our respiratory tracts. The functions of sinuses include humidifying air, providing cushioning for the skull and increasing the resonance of the voice.

There are four types of sinuses that surround the nose, called the *maxillary*, *frontal*, *sphenoid* and *ethmoid*. When each (or all)

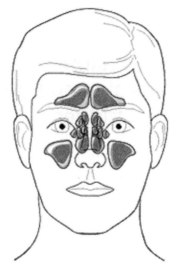

Figure 1.1 The sinuses

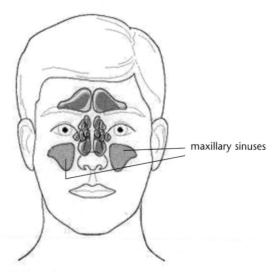

Figure 1.2 The maxillary sinuses

is inflamed from infection or allergic challenge different symptoms are experienced.

The shaded area in Figure 1.2 indicates the *maxillary* sinuses, located just behind the cheekbones on either side of the nose. If you have an inflammation of the maxillary sinuses you may experience:

- cheek pain/pressure
- toothache
- headaches

In Figure 1.3 the shaded area identifies the *frontal* sinuses, located just above the bone at the centre of each eyebrow. As with all of the other sinuses there is a ventilation/drainage tube between the inside of the nose and the frontal sinus. If you have an inflammation of the frontal sinuses you may experience:

- pain around and behind the eyes
- headaches

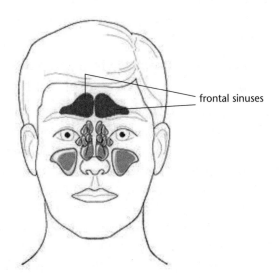

Figure 1.3 The frontal sinuses

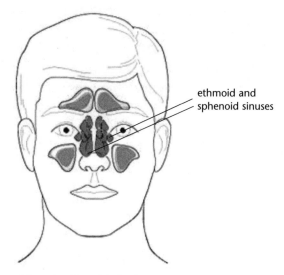

ethmoid and
sphenoid sinuses

Figure 1.4 The ethmoid and sphenoid sinuses

The shaded area in Figure 1.4 identifies the *ethmoid* and *sphenoid* sinuses. The ethmoid sinuses are located between the eyes and just behind the bridge of the nose. Behind the ethmoid sinuses, tucked in behind the eyes, are the sphenoid sinuses. If you have an inflammation of either or both you may experience:

- pain/pressure between and behind the eyes
- headaches

Barring injury and accidents, all sinus problems begin inside the nose. Sinuses can become inflamed, usually as a result of infection or allergic irritation, technically known as allergic challenge (there are other causes you can read about further on). When the internal lining of the nose swells (for whatever reason), the natural channel between nose and sinuses becomes obstructed. If the swelling persists then the sinus cavity stagnates. Air cannot flow freely in and out and the sinus lining also begins to swell. Tiny hair-like strands along the respiratory tract, called cilia, push mucus up towards our nose and mouth.

When the lining of the sinuses swells this mucus becomes stuck and causes uncomfortable pressure. It also produces a perfect breeding ground for bacteria.

So the first point to grasp is that sinusitis (inflammation and swelling of the delicate membranes that line the sinus cavities) starts only when swelling within the nose blocks the sinus openings, interfering with drainage and ventilation of the cavity. In turn this triggers sinus-lining swelling. Depending on how long this sequence continues, infection may set in and then all hell breaks loose. The discomfort experienced may feature some or all of the following:

- prolonged cold with a stuffy nose
- green, yellow or blood-streaked mucus coming from the nose
- pain in the head that worsens when lying down or bending over
- reduced sense of smell and taste
- reduced hearing
- bad breath
- copious drip of mucus down the back of the throat
- snoring
- sleep apnoea, where prolonged sleep deprivation is experienced throughout the night due to poor oxygen intake
- dry mouth from mouth breathing
- irritable, red eyes
- dark circles under the eyes
- puffy lower eyelids
- coughing and wheezing
- extreme fatigue to the point of exhaustion

In children there are the added problems of poor concentration, impaired hearing and general irritability, along with indifferent school performance. You can read more about this in Chapter 8.

Problems caused by sinusitis

The end result of persistent or recurring sinus problems is wide ranging. It can trigger a range of other problems, as set out below and explained in more detail throughout the book.

- There is an important link between the nose/sinuses and lungs. Infected or inflamed sinuses can trigger chest symptoms such as coughs, wheezing and shortness of breath.
- All asthma starts as an untreated nose and sinus irritation (see Chapter 4).
- All asthma involves problems in the nose and sinuses. If the nose and sinus issue is not treated then you will experience unnecessary extra discomfort and may have to use more anti-asthma medication than necessary.
- In aggressive nose and sinus swelling the Eustachian tube (the tiny tube at the back of the throat that connects with the inner ear) may become blocked. This can result in hearing loss, or at least reduced hearing acuity.
- Running along the 'ceiling' of the nose is a delicate nerve ending that transmits taste and smell to the brain. With persistent swelling of the nasal lining this nerve becomes so squeezed that it begins to lose its function. When this happens, the first sensation to fade is the sense of smell. After that the sense of taste, especially for spice, becomes impaired. Neglected, both taste and smell can be lost (but do recover with the correct treatment).
- Significant post-nasal drip can cause nausea and decreased appetite. This is an important factor in children, who may be frail and look undernourished.
- There is a nerve link between the nose and eyes such that an irritated nose eventually triggers irritable eyes.
- Significant nasal obstruction can cause heavy snoring. Sometimes the obstruction is so severe and the snoring so loud that the condition called sleep apnoea begins. This involves

recurring periods of total oxygen loss as the snorer struggles to get air through a very blocked nose, leading to such an impaired sleep pattern that the unfortunate person rarely wakens feeling refreshed. It also causes daytime drowsiness (some people have been known to fall asleep at their desks or even at the wheel of the car while driving). Long-term sleep apnoea in adults can put pressure on the cardiovascular system (see Chapter 9).

- Sleep apnoea in children causes fatigue, poor concentration, mood irritability and behavioural disturbances (there's more on this in Chapter 8).
- Adults and children with persisting or recurring sinus problems usually have a worsening of their symptoms during the changes of seasons in March/April and September/October. The September/October change causes most problems and starts with a 'head cold' that just won't go away.
- In aggressive, allergy-driven sinusitis there is often dramatic fluid blistering of the nose lining that further blocks the sinus openings.
- Sinusitis can be a trigger for migraine attacks.

Summary

As you can see, sinusitis is a very significant medical problem. To repeat, even at the risk of boring you: almost all sinus problems occur because of obstruction of the tubes connecting the nose to the inside of the sinuses. And almost all sinus problems can be helped by unblocking these tubes.

2

Types and causes of sinusitis

Types of sinusitis

Doctors divide sinus problems into different categories for ease of management:

1 Acute sinusitis (lasting up to four weeks).
2 Chronic sinusitis (lasting 12 weeks or more). People sometimes use the word 'chronic' to mean severe (as in 'I've got a chronic headache'). In medicine, 'chronic' means any condition lasting longer than 12 weeks.
3 Fungal sinusitis (this is a very important cause and one that researchers are studying in great detail. In the US some specialists believe as much as 90 per cent of long-standing sinusitis is due to fungal infection). There is more on this in Chapter 5.

Acute sinusitis

Acute sinusitis is usually the result of a virus 'head cold'. The nasal lining becomes swollen; there are runny nose symptoms with lots of handkerchiefs and paper tissues. Quite often people feel as if they've come down with the flu, get bad headaches and take to bed. They consume lots of hot drinks and usually some decongestant recommended by a pharmacist (or promoted on TV advertisements). It is big business and pharmaceutical companies set aside significant budgets for direct advertising to consumers.

If it's a true viral head cold it should be self-limiting and not drag on for more than a couple of weeks, with the nose and sinus lining eventually settling back to normal.

However, occasionally a 'head cold' can trigger significant swelling and inflammation of the nose and sinus linings. Then other bugs, especially bacteria, settle on the damaged tissue. That's when true sinusitis (sinus infection) kicks in and the symptoms become more aggressive with fever, pain and lethargy. A 14-day course of an antibiotic combined with an oral or 'direct-into-the-nose' decongestant will clear the problem.

Chronic sinusitis

Chronic sinusitis (with symptoms lasting longer than four weeks) tends to provoke more aggressive symptoms including fever, green or yellow nasal discharge, blurred vision and intense headache. Chronic sinusitis is complicated because there may be a number of interrelated causes – doctors call this *multi-factorial*. In plain English this suggests there may be a number of different triggers coming together at the same time to cause chaos. This is the 'perfect storm' of sinusitis. Allergy testing, blood testing, CT (computed tomography) scans, nasal endoscopies and acid-reflux studies (explained later in this chapter) are often used to clarify the situation.

Fungal sinusitis

Fungal sinusitis was once considered a rarity but may be more common than previously realized. Symptoms are often similar to those of bacterial sinusitis, except that the fungal infection may trigger fleshy (benign) growths inside the nose, called polyps. People who are allergic to fungi are often more susceptible to this particular form of sinusitis. A CT scan commonly determines whether or not a fungal infection has occurred, and standard procedures such as endoscopic surgery (see Chapter 3) are considered to clear the offended fungus and resume normal sinus drainage. Chapter 5 deals with fungal sinusitis in more detail.

Hazel

A 38-year-old IT consultant, for the past 12 months Hazel has been feeling sluggish, tired and lethargic a lot of the time. She has a constant headache that has become more of a nuisance in the past few months. She rarely wakens feeling refreshed and would nod off in front of her PC if it wasn't for the background babble of a busy open-plan office.

One of her friends comments on the amount of tissues filling Hazel's wastepaper bin. The same colleague wonders why Hazel seems to have a 'head cold' all the time. Now Hazel has a feel for her gradual and subtle loss of good health.

She makes an appointment with her family doctor, who examines Hazel from top to toe. When he inspects the internal lining of Hazel's nose he notices that the membrane is so swollen that it's obstructing her ability to breathe freely through the nose. He suspects Hazel cannot get a refreshing night's sleep because of this and suggests the explanation for her symptoms is a background sinusitis. Hazel is astonished – she never thought of herself as a sinus patient. 'What's causing this?' she asks. A battery of tests and sinus scans are arranged to answer Hazel's understandable question.

The scan shows considerable thickening of the sinuses on Hazel's forehead (frontal sinuses) as well as those on the side of her face (maxillary and ethmoid). It also confirms the doctor's observation about swelling of the nasal membrane. However, Hazel has no allergies so that cause is discounted.

Hazel smokes 20 cigarettes a day and has done for close on 15 years. Every January she kicks the habit and around mid-February her resolve breaks down and she lights up again. Hazel is also on an oral contraceptive pill. This is a dangerous combination in a 38-year-old woman. Hazel's age, combined with a high cigarette count and use of the contraceptive pill, puts her at risk of a heart attack, stroke or blood clot in the leg.

For these reasons alone she will have to change her lifestyle. But, as all other causes of her sinusitis have been discounted, the doctor concludes that the high number of cigarettes she has smoked over a long period, combined with her use of the contraceptive pill, have damaged her nose and sinus linings. Now Hazel is faced with a significant health issue. There are already signs of wear and tear in her nose and sinuses from cigarettes and taking the contraceptive pill. She is also at risk from other illnesses if she continues with this combination. But, her doctor reassures her, if she gives up the cigarettes and uses some other (non-hormonal) form of contraception, her good health can be restored.

She agrees to this (she really doesn't have any choice), and starts on a course of treatment for the nose and sinuses using special nasal decongestant drops and a follow-up nasal salt and baking soda irrigation product (all explained in subsequent chapters). Within a month her quality of life is dramatically improved and she feels reinvigorated. Six months later a follow-up sinus scan shows almost total clearance of the swollen lining inside the sinuses and nose.

Causes of chronic sinusitis

The following are the usual suspects responsible for chronic, i.e. ongoing, sinusitis. Not all relate to the same person, but quite often a combination of at least two or more cause sinus misery:

- Allergy, usually to inhaled allergy-provoking substances such as dust mites, moulds, pollens, animal hair, etc. Very rarely (and I do mean rarely), food allergy can cause sinus symptoms. You can read more on this in Chapter 11.
- Cigarette smoking (part of Hazel's downfall).
- Environmental irritants such as cement dust, laboratory fumes, ammonia dyes in hair dressing salons, etc..
- Atmospheric pollution.
- Poor air conditioning in your workplace.
- Bacterial infection.
- Fungal infection (read more on this in Chapter 5).
- Over-use of nasal decongestants.
- Dental problems. The roots of the upper posterior teeth are in close proximity to the maxillary sinus. If there is an infection at the root of one of these teeth, or under a crown in that area, it can spread to the adjoining sinus.
- Hormone changes in women. The menopause does cause significant nose and sinus irritability. So too can the oral contraceptive pill and hormone replacement therapy.
- Certain medications, especially aspirin, anti-arthritis and some blood pressure tablets.

- Structural defects that you might have been born with or acquired. These include abnormally narrow nose-to-sinus channels (you're born with these) or a bent nose due to the central cartilage in the nose, called the nasal septum, being crooked. You may have had this since childhood or acquired it through injury. If a structural defect is causing your problems, then only corrective surgery will allow you to lead a normal life. All the drugs in the world won't work – a surgical cure is vital.

- Cocaine abuse. This is an increasing problem for doctors dealing with sinusitis. Cocaine wears away the nasal lining and may even destroy the bony cartilage that separates one nostril from the other. Cocaine users have overly exaggerated symptoms. They complain bitterly about the pain and malaise of their 'sinusitis', the dramatic discomfort they experience, and that 'nothing I've been given helps'. Nothing will help (nor can help) while the cocaine abuse continues. Unfortunately coke heads have little insight in grasping the connection between their poor health and drug addiction. They deny any link when it's pointed out. 'I haven't done coke for a month and my sinuses have been awful for the past week.' Apart from wearing out their nose and sinuses, these people wear out the patience of the treating doctor.

Gerry

Successful accountant Gerry earns good money, is single and lives in an apartment. He likes the good life and is a 'recreational' drug user. His favourite night out is a few beers in the pub, wine with an Indian or Chinese meal and then off to a night-club to party. He'll probably smoke a few joints en route and snort cocaine in the toilets. He may even take an 'E' to keep the party mood flowing. However Gerry's behaviour is becoming increasingly erratic: he's prone to mood swings, is easily angered and seems to have a constant head cold. He complains bitterly that his GP can't do anything for him and that even an ENT specialist was 'useless'. Inevitably Gerry's lifestyle catches up with him: after a heavy night of drink and drugs he falls, bangs his head and is taken to A&E. He is semi-conscious and disorientated, his speech slurred: the doctors decide to keep him in for investigation. They fear he has suffered a serious head injury. Blood tests reveal high levels of alcohol, amphetamines and cocaine in his blood. Special scans show no injury to the brain but considerable damage to the nose and sinuses. Gerry is referred to a rehab unit but fails to keep his appointment. Gerry will party until he drops dead or throws himself off a high building believing he can fly. The UK and Ireland have plenty of Gerrys and the number is growing.

Investigating the triggers

So how do doctors know which trigger or combination of triggers is causing sinusitis?

Commonly they decide on the basis of how the symptoms began (called 'the history'). They will ask some of the following questions to get more information.

1 How long is it since you were last fully well?
2 How did the sinusitis start, slowly or suddenly?
3 Do you have any idea what brought it on in the first place or makes it worse now?
4 What have you found helpful in giving you relief so far?
5 What have you tried that didn't make any difference, or even made you feel worse?
6 Have you been using a lot of non-prescription nasal decongestants?
7 How is your general health?
8 Do you have any background medical condition that may be irritating your nose and sinuses?
9 Are you on any medication that might trigger nose and sinus problems?
10 Is there a family history of nose and/or sinus problems?
11 Do you snore?
12 Do you mouth breathe while asleep?
13 Do you get a lot of post-nasal drip?
14 Do you suffer heartburn?
15 Is your sense of smell or taste impaired?

16 Do you break out in hives (intensely itchy skin bumps, called *urticaria* by doctors)?

17 Have you ever had an allergic reaction to aspirin/dispirin or other painkillers?

18 Does Indian or Chinese or Oriental food make you feel unwell or bring you out in itchy bumps (there's more on this in Chapter 9)?

19 Do you have asthma or do you get 'chesty' each time your sinuses act up?

The answer to these gives a valuable insight into the type of sinus problem you may have.

Next there is a general physical examination to make sure the sinusitis isn't merely one of a group of features of certain conditions.

In most specialized sinusitis centres an *allergy test* is now performed. This is done by the 'skin-prick test' format. With a skin-prick test the doctor places a concentrated drop of allergy extract on to the skin (usually the forearm but occasionally the back, especially in small children). Each drop contains a test substance such as dust mite, cat hair, horsehair, grass pollen or specific foods.

The surface of the skin is rich in mast cells. To cut through a lot of unnecessary medical jargon, these cells recognize what you are allergic to. The test drop is brought into direct contact with the skin mast cells by pricking the surface and allowing the fluid to seep to a lower level. If you are allergic to a specific substance the mast cells underneath will 'explode' and a reaction appears. The size of the central blister plus any surrounding skin redness tells the doctor what you are allergic to, and how strongly allergic.

The final interpretation depends on symptoms, what the doctor discovers when he examines your nose and sinuses and what reactions come up on testing. There is more about skin-prick allergy testing, and other allergy tests, in Chapter 11.

Probably a range of blood tests will be arranged at this point to check your general health and offer insights into any background ailments that might produce sinus-type symptoms. For example, immune disorders, including the inability to manufacture the cells that fight infection (antibodies), are occasionally a cause of persisting sinusitis. The final interpretation here can include monitoring your body's ability to make antibodies after vaccination. Some centres treat people with reduced immunity with intravenous gamma-globulin antibody therapy. This boosts their immunity and ability to fight infection.

This is now followed by direct inspection of the nose using a simple light source (much the same sort of instrument that doctors use to look in people's ears). However this gives only a limited view of the nose and sinuses. More commonly a flexible fibre optic (such as the Olympus ENF fibrescope, shown in Figure 2.1 overleaf) with a camera chip attached is inserted into the nose and threaded all the way to the vocal cords. The fibrescope is no more than 3 mm in diameter, so it passes easily and painlessly. The state of the nose and all structures within the nose can be seen and recorded. The sinus openings can be observed. The doctor can spot infected material oozing from the sinuses, or identify abnormalities within the bony structure of the nose. The state of the tissue at the back of the throat can be checked and any post-nasal drip noted. The adenoid, tonsils and vocal cords can be viewed. The adenoid is spongy tissue at the back of the throat in children up to the age of 12 years that can be so large it interferes with the function of the nose and developing sinuses. Dramatic and detailed fibre-optic images can be viewed on <www.allergy-ireland.ie>, 'Dedicated sinusitis facility'.

The usefulness of this instrument cannot be underestimated as it allows your doctor to have a better understanding of what you are complaining about, and the likely causes.

Special X-rays, called CT scans, may be ordered to give a clearer picture of what's happening in the sinuses. CT scans

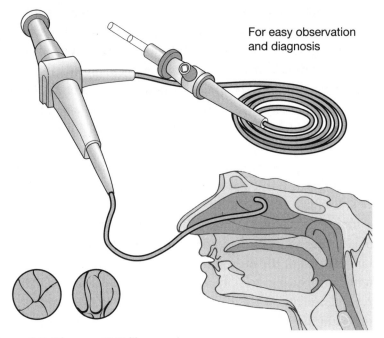

For easy observation and diagnosis

Figure 2.1 Olympus ENF fibrescope

highlight the soft membranes of the sinuses and show damage, infection or the presence of the fleshy soft tissue swellings called polyps. There is a significant amount of exposure to radiation with CT scan imaging, so don't expect your treating doctor to order this at the drop of a tissue. Also, the scans are expensive and healthcare budgetary restraints may dictate whether they are reserved only for very ill people.

Finally, where there is any suspicion of stomach acid reflux (your doctor is likely to investigate this if you answered 'yes' to the heartburn question, although some individuals do have reflux without symptoms), an evaluation of the stomach and gullet may be ordered. This may take the form of a gastroscopy (a flexible fibre optic passed directly into the stomach via the gullet) or a barium-swallow X-ray. Here a radioactive dye (barium) is swallowed and its passage through the gullet and stomach is captured on X-ray. This may show significant spilling-back of stomach acid contents towards the nose and sinuses, thus irritating their delicate lining. Diet plus special anti-reflux drugs often cure this situation.

Post-nasal drip, without other symptoms of sinusitis, is often caused by acid reflux.

Summary

With persisting sinus symptoms, your treating doctor will try and get to the bottom of all potential causes before he or she selects a treatment course. There's no point in shoving drugs at you until he or she has a handle on background trigger(s). Also, treatments are tailored to cause. What might work for allergic sinusitis will not make a blind bit of difference with infected sinusitis. Fungal sinusitis may respond to antifungal treatments, whereas hormone-induced sinus problems require a completely different strategy.

It may sound complicated but in practice it's fairly straightforward. So let's move on to the next chapter and discuss treatment options.

3

Treating sinusitis

Almost all sinus problems begin inside the nose.

Every working day in my clinic people relate how miserable their lives are since they developed sinus problems. Sometimes they are children as young as five (although young children's sinuses may not be fully developed, they can still get significant problems inside the nose). Since children cannot always vocalize how they feel it's up to their parents to describe the ill-health.

'He's constantly stuffed up in the nose.'

'He's always complaining of headaches. It's going on so long we had him checked for a brain tumour. Thankfully that was clear but he still whines about headaches, especially around the forehead.'

'She won't stop rubbing and picking at her nose.'

'He's sniffling and snorting all the time and it's driving the rest of us mad. He just doesn't seem to know how to blow his nose.'

'I'm buying Kleenex her/him like it's going out of fashion. His pockets are bulging with snotty, bunched up tissues.'

'He's exhausted and he's got big dark circles round his eyes.'

And those are some of the more generous descriptions and comments.

Often the child is also grumpy, irritable, moody and out of sorts. Those features are usually mentioned by way of handwritten notes so the parents' concerns aren't talked about in front of the child. They wonder if this is the boy or girl's true temperament, or simply his or her response to ill-health.

With adults the complaints are up front and loud. There's no holding back or couching the language in subtle tones.

'I feel absolutely awful.'

'I'm miserable. It's like I have a constant flu bug.'

'I'm not sleeping properly and my wife says I snore so loud she can't sleep either. When I wake up in the morning my mouth feels dry because I'm breathing through it all night.'

'Help!'

With all people, adults or children, I have a strategy to identify what the real issue is, how to explain it and then how to put things right. So pretend you're in my clinic and let me set out my stall of management.

In the clinic

First I listen carefully to the complaints, trying not to interrupt so I get a feel for the severity of the symptoms and how they are affecting the person concerned.

Next I pose leading questions so as to understand better what's likely to be going on in the nose and sinuses. I may quiz the person about snoring and mouth breathing, about loss of taste and smell, about mucus flow down the back of the throat, about headaches or pain along the upper teeth and gums, about coughing and wheezing and shortness of breath (all of which can be present in children as well as adults). Then I ask whether the person (or the parent) knows of any obvious triggers that might make the symptoms worse (or better). Does anyone in the household smoke (the person or parent)? What about passive smoking? I check about long-term medicines and general health, and I ask for honesty about drug abuse, especially cocaine.

Now I inspect the nasal cavity (in other words I shine a very bright light up the nose and examine all the structures that can be observed). This gives an instant impression of what the problem is. Then, using a flexible fibrescope, I inspect the nasal lining from nose tip to throat. As the fibrescope moves along,

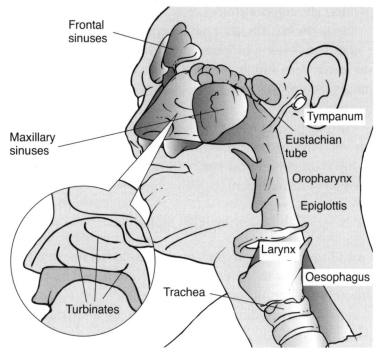

Figure 3.1 The nose, throat and sinuses

an exact image is captured on an LCD screen. I can then point out what the problem is and the patient or parent can see exactly the cause behind the unwellness. Often the images are so dramatic that the person (and especially the parent) is quite shocked at the final picture.

At this point I explain the connection between symptoms and what I've spotted with the fibrescope. Using a diagram of the nose and sinuses like that shown in Figure 3.1, I describe their function and interconnection.

I use words like these: 'The lining of the nose is delicate and easily damaged. Running along the inside are three shelf-like structures called *turbinates*. These clean, filter, warm and moisten the air we breathe before it enters the lungs. But the turbinates are easily injured. Ignoring physical trauma, any challenge that aggressively irritates the nasal lining may cause the turbinates to swell. The challenge can range from infection, to allergy, to cigarette smoking, to inhaling chemical vapours, etc. When the turbinates swell they block the little tubes that drain the sinuses into the nose. Now we not only have a nose problem but the beginning of sinusitis.'

Almost all sinus problems begin inside the nose.

'If the swelling within the nose persists,' I continue, 'the sinuses cannot breathe, their air pockets stagnate and become a rich feeding ground for infection with viruses, moulds and bacteria. There is a link between the nose and sinuses, so unchecked sinusitis and rhinitis (the medical term for nose irritability) can cause coughing, wheezing and breathing difficulties.'

I let that sink in for a minute. 'Running along the ceiling of the nose is an exquisitely delicate nerve ending that transmits the sensations of taste and smell to the brain. With prolonged pressure on this nerve from turbinate swelling these sensations fade.

'So,' I go on, 'when you say you think you have a sinus problem, quite often you're missing the connection between the swelling inside your nose and the back pressure it creates on the surrounding sinuses. I cannot make the sinuses better without first restoring the nose to normal.'

'And how can we do that?' I'm asked.

'Simple,' I say, 'we use special unblocking drops, safe for adults and children when prescribed correctly. The only difficulty (and it's not significant) is that the drops have to be taken in a special "head-back" or "head-forward" position.'

Using unblocking drops

Figure 3.2 shows how the drops are used. The person lies on a couch or bed so that the head can bend to a 90-degree angle, either forwards or backwards. *Children really only benefit from*

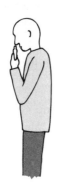

Bend head forward and hold chin in.

Hold the spray in the left hand to treat right nostril and vice versa.

If using squirts, alter the angle to wet as much as possible of the inside of the nostril.

Do not sniff too hard as this drags the solution too quickly to the back of the throat.

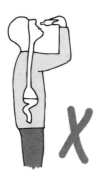

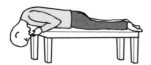 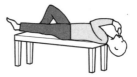

Figure 3.2 How to use nose drops and nose spray

the head-back, rather than the head-forward strategy. The idea is to allow the prescribed drops (called Betnesol, chemical name betamethasone) to trickle around the swollen nose lining, coat all the tissue and find a resting point at the 'ceiling' level of the nose. The medicine in Betnesol slowly reduces the swollen nasal and turbinate linings. How long the drops are used depends on how blocked the nose is at the start of treatment. Typically therapy can vary from between five days in small children to three or even four weeks in adults.

When the nose is sufficiently unblocked, a nose spray is used to stabilize the nasal cavity. The spray (and there are a number of excellent products) is directed into the now normal-looking nose in a dosage decided by your treating doctor. The purpose is to maintain the improvement that we've achieved with the Betnesol drops. If we just treat with drops and stop as soon as normality is achieved, unfortunately the nasal lining may swell again. So it's very important not only to restore the nose to health but keep it unblocked.

Betnesol nose drops: how to use them correctly

Here's a typical regime for an adult:

- Get into the position suggested (see Figure 3.2).
- Instil two drops into each nostril (it might be easier to have someone help you with this, as it's not easy to concentrate on the correct position *and* ensure you're getting the drops in properly).
- Stay in the position for three minutes.
- After three minutes pinch the soft part of your nose closed. Now lift your head to the normal position (some drops may spill out at this point, but that's not important).
- Do this twice daily (preferably morning and evening) for 14 days.
- On Day 15 start the nasal spray (Nasacort or Flixonase or Avamys or Nasonex: these are the trade names for a group of excellent nose sprays used in persistent sinusitis). The dosage is one squiff up into each nostril (as shown in Figure 3.2) twice daily. Continue this until you see your doctor again.
- In the meantime (or at any time in the future where this is an ongoing programme), if you get breakthrough 'head cold' symptoms, stop the spray and restart the Betnesol drops (administering them in the same position as shown in Figure 3.2) until the blockage clears. This may take as little as one to two days. Even if it takes longer, persist. The nasal spray cannot work if you are spraying it into a blocked/runny nose. The aim of this plan is to restore the nose and sinuses to their normal function.
- Don't worry if there isn't total control, some fine-tuning may be necessary until the treatment takes full effect.

If the background cause is allergy driven (almost always through breathing in allergic substances such as dust mites, pollen and animal hair – see Chapter 11), and especially if there are associated chest problems such as coughing and wheezing, then oral anti-allergy medicines, either Singulair (chemical name montelukast) or Accolate (chemical name zafirlukast), may be added. These compounds, called *leukotriene receptor antagonists*, block one of the most important chemicals involved in nose, sinus and chest allergy. They work just as well in nose and sinus allergy that doesn't involve the chest.

If the sinusitis is a reasonably recent event and associated, say, with high pollen counts, then an antihistamine would be a better alternative than Singulair or Accolate. Go for one of the newer, non-drowsy products such as Xyzal (levocetrizine), Zirtek (cetrizine) or Neoclarityn (desloratadine).

To minimize the amount of medicine required for long-term control, I strongly recommend nasal douching (explained in detail in Chapter 12). This involves irrigating the nasal passages with a warm water solution of salt and baking soda. This clears any dirt, snot, crud, mucus, crusting, dry blood, etc. that tends to collect in stubborn nose and sinus problems. Go for the Neilmed brand of sinus rinse. It's a winner for all types of sinusitis: allergic, non-allergic, chemically irritated, etc.

Using unblocking drops: questions and answers

This all sounds too easy. Will it work?
Yes. Failure of treatments is usually due to incorrect use of drops, not taking them long enough or failing to follow through with the nose spray immediately after the course of drops. If there is a deep infection within the sinuses, that too will block progress and a prolonged course of an antibiotic will be needed. One other consideration is if the bony structure of the nose is crooked: then there is an anatomical abnormality that must be

put right and no medication can do that. There's more on this below.

What's in the Betnesol drops?
Cortisone (a steroid). This is the only medication that will successfully shrink the swollen and distorted nasal lining back to normal. Provided you stick to the recommended dose you need not fear side-effects. Cortisone can produce problems such as weight gain, facial bloating, sleeplessness and mood swings, but with the strategy suggested here none should occur. If you have any concerns, check with your family doctor for advice. Equally, do not self-medicate with Betnesol drops without keeping your treating doctor informed. He or she needs to know how much and how often you're taking this medication because there is a point at which side-effects might occur. (One of the many reasons I'm a big fan of nasal douching is that it keeps the nasal/sinus linings clean and fresh and less likely to break down again and again. Daily nasal douching should allow you to keep prescribed medicines to a minimum. And it's only a salt and baking soda mixture, totally harmless but very effective.)

What's in the nose sprays?
Cortisone (a steroid). Again, this is the only medicine that successfully stabilizes and protects the nose and sinus linings, especially when the problem is allergy driven. The nose sprays have exact doses in each 'squiff' so it's actually quite difficult to overdose on them. Regular use does not damage the nose, thin the nose lining, make the nose lining more vulnerable to infections (or any other scare story you've heard about them). Nor does the medication get absorbed into the blood circulation when used according to the prescriber's instructions.

Does this strategy work for all types of sinusitis? Is it as effective in allergic as non-allergic sinusitis? What about chemically irritated sinusitis, or hormone-related sinusitis, or stomach acid reflux sinusitis?

The core principle of dealing with any type of sinusitis is to restore the nasal lining to normal first. Whatever the cause, the nose must be unblocked to allow the sinuses to breathe again. So the Betnesol drops plan is for all types of sinusitis. Working on the background causes is important, of course, but the nose must be normalized at the same time.

What if this plan doesn't work?
I'm assuming all background causes have been addressed, any coexisting infection cleared and prescribed treatments followed religiously. If all that fails, now we're looking at surgery.

Surgical treatments for sinusitis

Surgery in sinusitis is used for five main reasons:

1 To correct any anatomical deformity (such as a significantly crooked septum, the cartilage that separates one nostril from the other) or widen any abnormally narrow drainage tubes between nose and sinuses.
2 To remove any abnormal swellings or growths (such as nose polyps – see Chapter 6). By clearing the nasal cavity of all obstructions, surgery allows good sinus drainage again.
3 To deal with any stubborn infection that is not responding to adequate medical therapy. Here the commonest procedure is called functional endoscopic sinus surgery (FESS). This is a minimally invasive technique (in other words it's a delicate and deliberate surgical skill, there's no brute force and ignorance employed!) to restore sinus ventilation and normal function. Fibre-optic telescopes are used for diagnosis and during the procedure a CT scan assesses the anatomy and identifies diseased areas. FESS is reserved for when medical treatment has failed. The procedure can be performed under general or local anaesthesia on an outpatient basis with little discomfort.

4 To deal with any aggressive infection which, despite even intravenous antibiotic therapy, is obviously spreading. There's a golden rule in medicine: where there's pus collecting, drain it.

5 To debulk the nasal lining where it is swollen, obstructing and just not budging despite the best medical therapies. The introduction of the microdebrider in the early 1990s helped to popularize this approach. This electrically powered instrument shaves away and removes diseased tissue, one thin layer at a time, leaving the healthy lining unharmed. Quick healing usually follows this gentle surgical technique.

Image-guided sinus surgery is used in some specialized sinusitis surgery centres. During the procedure, the surgeon interacts with three-dimensional CT images on a powerful computer system, attached to the person via a headset. With this perspective, the surgeon can positively pinpoint areas of disease as well as maintain the ideal positioning of surgical instruments in the person's complex and delicate sinus cavities, providing a real-time surgical road map. This image-guided technique dramatically improves surgical accuracy, leading to more consistent results, and shortened operating and anaesthesia time.

A new technique, *balloon sinuplasty*, uses inflatable balloon tipped catheters to dilate narrowed sinus openings, without removal of any tissues. This is similar to the procedures used in cardiac catheterization and is appropriate in certain cases.

Minimally invasive, targeted surgical techniques are now widely recognized as the most effective, least discomforting and least invasive approach to remedying sinus disease. *However, when all is said and done, sinusitis is mainly a medical problem and surgery is the treatment of last resort.*

Summary

- If your house is on fire, put the flames out first and then ask how it happened and what do you do to stop it happening again. With persisting sinusitis, first get better and then decide what the background cause is. Finally, work on a long-term strategy to keep your sinuses healthy.
- Almost all sinus problems begin inside the nose. Keep your nose healthy and your sinuses will stay healthy too.
- The degree of swelling and obstruction within the nasal cavity determines how long it takes to recover sinus health.
- In some conditions of the nose and sinuses, especially when the trigger is an allergy to airborne allergens such as dust mites, grass pollens, etc., not only does the nose lining swell but it blisters from fluid bubbling underneath the surface.
- The first stage of management involves unblocking the nose with Betnesol drops. The second stage involves stabilizing the nose and sinuses with a nasal spray.
- For allergic nose and sinus problems that may be stubborn to settle, a course of steroid tablets will often produce the final clearance.
- If medical treatments fail to clear your sinus problems then surgery is almost certainly your best option.
- Nasal douching (see Chapter 12) with a salt and baking soda combination such as Neilmed Sinus Rinse keeps the nasal cavity clean and refreshed.
- Learn to treat your nose and sinuses with the same respect you would your teeth. Nasal hygiene is as important as dental hygiene for people with sinusitis.

4

Sinusitis, asthma and aspirin allergy

Let's start this chapter with a bit of controversy. In fact, let's be *very* controversial. There's no such thing as asthma. I'll rephrase that. There is a condition still called asthma, but it's now better incorporated into the term *united airways disease* (and no, that's not a low fares airline ailment!). United airways disease implies that asthma is but the *lung* component of a much more complicated condition that involves the nose, sinuses, lungs and bloodstream.

Harriet

Harriet, a 33-year-old publishing editor, had an intractable cough. She also had asthma and was using standard full strength anti-asthma therapy. The cough was socially embarrassing and spoiled her quality of life. Any type of conversation was cut short by a bout of convulsive spluttering. She attended two GPs in the same London practice and the respiratory unit of a top London teaching hospital. There she was reviewed by three specialists (one a pulmonary allergist), had multiple tests including chest X-ray, pulmonary function tests and allergy tests. She showed very strong responses to dust mites, pollens and cat hair. She was given a fact sheet on dust mites and de-cluttered her apartment to little more than bare boards and a wooden bed. Her cough continued. The hospital advised that nothing else could be done and suggested to her GP that this was possibly a psychological cough, recommending a mild tranquillizer. In desperation (and convinced it was not a psychological cough) she sought help elsewhere.

During questioning at a reputable private allergy clinic she agreed that her nose was blocked all the time, that her senses of taste and smell were poor and that her hearing had deteriorated ('I have had to turn up the volume on my iPod recently'). When examined she was found to have severe swelling of her nose lining with fluid blistering of the turbinates (the shelves along the nose – see Chapter 3). 'You're the first doctor to have inspected my nose,' she remarked. There was fluid behind both eardrums, suggesting Eustachian tube obstruction (see Chapter 1). Further questioning revealed that she worked in a smoky office (the smoking ban hadn't then come into effect in the UK in small offices) and that the owner had a large cat that shed hair.

It was explained that her cough was almost certainly due to her aggressive, unrecognized and untreated nose and sinus allergy. It was suggested that while her home environment might be perfect, her workplace was a definite health hazard. She was treated appropriately and her nasal cavity stabilized. To say her life changed for the better is an understatement: symptom scores for her sinusitis symptoms and asthma dropped by 80 per cent. The cough flared at work and in smoky environments, so she quit her job and found a better (and safer) office. Now she is enjoying a dramatically improved lifestyle. Her hearing has improved as well. However, she's quite annoyed with the NHS and that top London teaching hospital (not to mention her smoking colleagues and the boss's cat).

If an Oxford-educated (as Harriet is), articulate and successful publishing executive can have so much difficulty having her problem identified and treated, it says a lot about the continuing ignorance throughout the medical profession concerning the link between sinusitis and asthma. And its correct management.

Here are a few facts:

- Allergic sinusitis involves the nose as well as the sinuses.
- Allergic sinusitis may cause nose and sinus symptoms only.
- Allergic sinusitis may provoke chest symptoms as well.
- Allergic sinusitis may coexist with asthma.
- Allergic sinusitis, if left untreated, may allow nasal polyps to develop (see Chapter 6).
- Coexistent allergic sinusitis in asthmatic children causes them more asthma-related hospital admissions and greater total days spent in hospital than children who do not have the combination of sinusitis and asthma.

Links between sinusitis and asthma

The relationship between allergic sinusitis and asthma has been known about for some time (though listening to some doctors you might find that hard to believe) and people commonly come to their doctor with both disorders. Experts believe allergic sinusitis and asthma are connected by a number of different pathways. For example, post-nasal drip may contain cells that slip into the lungs and trigger asthma-type symptoms. Also, special blood units (called Th2) move from the nose and sinuses to the bone marrow to produce a number of allergy groupings. They then transfer into the blood circulation and 'stick' in the nose, sinuses and lungs, causing further allergic inflammation (swelling and irritability of the tissues involved). I appreciate this is all very complicated and medical (and to be honest, I'm not sure I understand the half of it myself, but I do recognize the sense behind the theory). The bottom line is this: treat the affected nose and sinuses and you improve any coexisting asthma significantly.

All children with true asthma also have some type of sinusitis, usually allergy-driven. When allergic sinusitis is very active, airway irritability increases, often aggravating the symptoms of asthma. Furthermore, the onset of allergic sinusitis sometimes precedes asthma and the onset of asthma may be prevented by successful treatment of allergic sinusitis.

Significant problems in the upper airways (i.e. the nose and sinuses) can produce symptoms in the lower respiratory tract (i.e. the lungs). Treat the upper respiratory problems and you can alleviate or even *cure* the lower respiratory trouble.

Patrick

Seven-year-old Patrick has troublesome asthma. He's seen many doctors, including asthma specialists, and is on a lot of anti-asthma medication. But he's still troubled with his chest and each breakdown in well-being seems to start with a head cold. There is a strong history of allergy in the family (two sisters had eczema as babies, his father has hay fever each summer) but no attention is paid to Patrick's parents' request for allergy testing ('waste of time, could be anything, try lifting the carpets', are the dismissive comments). Each doctor has advised that the boy had difficult asthma made worse by repeated virus infections. Live with it, they said. Stop annoying us, they didn't say but implied.

When Patrick was evaluated at a reputable allergy centre a completely different interpretation was put on his ill-health and its management. The examining doctor inspected the inside lining of Patrick's nose ('no other doctor has ever done that,' commented Patrick's mother). It was obvious Patrick had a severe nose and sinus allergy (swollen, pale and blistered nose lining, dramatic 'allergy-attack' features at the highest point of his nose). He was wheezing loudly despite taking his prescribed anti-asthma therapy.

Allergy testing revealed strong positives to dust mites and cat hair (the family had a pet cat and it often slept on Patrick's bed).

His new management included an aggressive anti-allergy regime (full details in Chapter 11), restoring his nasal membrane to normal and stabilizing with a nose spray (as set out in Chapter 3). Because Patrick had both nose and sinus and lung allergic challenges he was prescribed the anti-allergy drug Singulair. For the first time in years Patrick's quality of life improved. He showed a dramatic recovery in his chest as his nose and sinus problems came under control. After about four weeks his asthma medication was reduced by as much as 80 per cent.

Patrick now has excellent asthma control with fewer drugs being used. And he feels much more comfortable in his 'head', now that his nose is unblocked and his sinuses function properly.

What can we conclude from this? Patrick's upper airways allergy (sinusitis) was impacting on his lower airways (lungs, causing asthma). Once identified and treated, Patrick's out-of-control allergic sinusitis changed the boy's life for ever. And his parents weren't half pleased too.

This is not a textbook (as I've said elsewhere) and I do not propose to quote chapter and verse and every reference to support this concept. However it's now recognized internationally that asthma is but one component of a more complex and complicated interreaction of nose/sinus problems and the lungs. It's a real shame that chest specialists don't inspect the nose and sinuses as part of their overall assessment of people suspected of having asthma. Equally, it's quite frustrating for people to attend ear, nose and throat specialists who will never check their very obvious coughs and wheezes. It's almost as if they're afraid to make the connection. (Or add to their workload? It's easy to be cynical here.)

To sum up:

- All asthma probably begins in the nose and sinuses and then spreads to involve the lungs.
- Asthma as a solo lung condition probably doesn't exist, there's almost always some degree of nose and sinus involvement. Treating asthma alone without addressing the associated nose and sinus problems condemns you to unnecessary anti-asthma drugs and misses the focal point of where the problem lies.
- Doctors should always inspect the nose and sinuses as part of their assessment of adults and children with asthma. Doctors should deal properly with the associated nose and sinus issues when considering how to help their asthmatic patients.

It isn't rocket science. It's more important than rocket science. It could be you or your child suffering needlessly.

Sinusitis and aspirin allergy

Now we have agreed on the link between sinusitis and asthma I have one more piece of information to share with you. And it's very important.

Between 30 and 40 per cent (the statistics vary according to which expert you ask, but let's use these figures as a reasonable guide) of asthmatics with chronic (ongoing) sinusitis will become seriously allergic to aspirin/Disprin at some stage in their lives. This means that if they take an aspirin or Disprin they will get an aggressive flare-up of their nose, sinus and chest symptoms. Occasionally this can be life-threatening. More commonly the reactions range from itchy hives to large swellings all over the body. Occasionally the face, lips and eyes swell to such an extent that the person looks like the 'Michelin Man'.

However the presence of aspirin is not always obvious. It is in many across-the-counter painkillers as well as various sinus tablets, medicines used to control period pain, and cold and flu tablets. If you are sensitive to aspirin, you will need to read medicine labels carefully and be cautious about taking any analgesic without talking to your doctor or pharmacist first. Here are some examples of what might contain aspirin:

- cold and flu tablets
- Alka-Seltzer
- period pain and headache tablets
- inflammatory bowel disease drugs, for example Mesalal and Salazopyrin
- complementary alternative medicines: willow tree bark extract, some herbal arthritis pills
- teething gels (Bonjela, Oral-sed gel)

However the situation is a little more complicated than this. The chemical name for aspirin is *sodium salicylate*. Salicylates occur naturally in certain foods and depending on your medical condition you may be told to avoid these totally, or, more likely, advised to consume them in small quantities only. Do not mix and match throughout this group such that you might unwittingly consume large quantities. The following foods all contain salicylates:

- dried fruits
- berry fruits
- oranges
- apricots
- pineapples
- cucumbers
- gherkins
- tomato sauce
- tea
- endives

- olives
- grapes
- almonds
- liquorice
- peppermints
- honey
- Worcester sauce

Many spices also contain high salicylate levels.

There's more. I apologize for this apparent information overload but it's better to learn these facts reading this book than hearing about them in the intensive care unit of your local hospital.

Some people with sinusitis have poor senses of smell and taste (if they were treated properly this wouldn't happen, but that's another day's work). When taste becomes impaired the sensation of spice is the first to go. So these people (adults and children) look for more tangy, spicier foods and flavourings. Unfortunately almost all tang and spice is artificially created using chemicals. And the compounds involved are not a million miles different in their chemical structure from aspirin. People can unwittingly make their sinus condition worse (and add in an extra problem) by using artificially flavoured foods, especially in Indian and Chinese dishes.

There are many chemical additives used by the food and drink industry and by law the manufacturer must inform the consumer what compounds are in the can or tin or packet. The additives are used to colour, flavour or preserve food and drinks. For example, if you buy a packet of 'cheese & onion' crisps, there's neither cheese nor onion in the product: the taste is created by a chemical. When you reach for a brightly coloured fizzy drink on the supermarket shelf, more often than not the colour is artificially created by a chemical. Some foods and drinks have all three types of chemicals in them: colourings, flavourings and preservatives. Because the chemicals have long and strange sounding names the industry works to a code. Nowadays each additive is labelled by number and with the letter E attached (known as 'E numbers').

So, as part of your overall management, you should avoid the following food additives (E number and original chemical name included):

- E122 (tartrazine)
- E104 (quinoline yellow)
- E107 (yellow 2G)
- E110 (sunset yellow)
- E122 (azorubine)
- E123 (amaranth)
- E124 (ponceau 4R)
- E127 (erythrosine)
- E128 (red 2G)
- E131 (patent blue)
- E132 (indigo carmine)
- E120–E219 inclusive (called the benzoates)
- E621, E622 and E623 (called the glutamates)

Especially look out for E621, monosodium glutamate, which is a widely used flavouring in snack foods, savouries, gravy mixes, stock cubes, packet/tinned soups, Indian, Chinese and Oriental foods, etc.

Where there is poor labelling, or the phrase 'contains permitted additives' or 'contains permitted colourings and flavourings', or just 'colourings and flavourings', avoid the product. Indeed avoid any product coloured red, orange, yellow, blue, lemon or green as there is a strong chance it may contain one of the listed agents. Check tablets, capsules, lozenges, vitamin preparations and even the stripes in toothpaste. If you are unsure about the safety of the product, avoid it.

Finally, there is a group of drugs called NSAIDs that are widely used by doctors for pain relief, to reduce fever, ease aches/

sprains, etc. (NSAID is short for non-steroidal anti-inflammatory drugs, in other words medicines that reduce inflammation and pain but do not contain any steroids or cortisone.) NSAIDs are also used in arthritis treatments and are produced as tablets, capsules, gel rubs and injections.

If you are allergic to aspirin/disprin you could also react to one of these drugs.

Do not allow a doctor to prescribe any of these compounds. Especially do not allow one of them to be administered by injection.

It would be wiser to endure the pain rather than experience a severe allergic reaction. There is a wide range of alternative pain-relieving drugs, including the popular and well known paracetamol compound.

The number of NSAIDs changes regularly as new drugs replace older products and it is very difficult keeping this list up to date. If in doubt, ask your pharmacist. However, the following should be avoided:

Alrheumat	Distamine	Lederfen	Palaprin
Ananase	Dolobid	Mefac	Ponalgic
Arthrotec	Feldene	Melfen	Ponmel
Ascriptin	Fenomel	Mesalal	Ponstan
Benoral	Fenopron	Methrazone	Progesic
Brufen	Flamrase	Mobiflex	Relifex
Bufigen	Flexin	Napmel	Rheumox
Caprin	Froben	Naprex	Salazoprin
Cidomel	Genoxon	Naprosyn	Surgam
Clinoril	Gerinap	Nuseals	Synflex
Codafen	Geroxican	Orudis	Tolectin
Cunil	Idomed	Orugesic	Vologen
Diclac	Imbrilon	Oruvail	Voltarol
Diclomel	Indocid	Perican	
Difene	Indomod	Pinalgesic	

This list may be incomplete, so check with your doctor or pharmacist if you have any doubts. *Many of these are available without prescription.*

Danny

Danny, 46, has a 20-year history of nose polyps (see Chapter 6), asthma and aspirin allergy. He's been cautioned that some painkilling drugs (known as anti-inflammatory compounds) are also dangerous. Danny is extremely careful about medication, always double-checking the ingredients of prescribed and over-the-counter products.

One day Danny strained his back at work. The company doctor examined him and decided he could be back on the production line quicker if he gave him an anti-inflammatory injection. Danny challenged the doctor three times about the ingredients of the injection. Three times he cautioned the doctor about his aspirin allergy and the possibility of anti-inflammatory injections triggering a dangerous reaction if prescribed, especially if injected. Three times the examining doctor played down Danny's fears, muttering at one stage that he didn't believe in 'all this allergy nonsense'. He gave Danny a 75 milligram injection of Diclofenac, a well-known, cheap and fast acting anti-inflammatory. Unfortunately it is on the list of banned compounds for those with an aspirin allergy.

Within minutes Danny felt unwell. His chest tightened, he started sweating. After around six minutes, he was experiencing his worst asthma attack ever and had gone blue. And the treating doctor was outside and about to drive off. By ten minutes Danny had collapsed, was gasping for air, restless and incoherent. The doctor rushed back in, took one look and (fortunately) realized what he'd done. He gave Danny an injection of adrenaline (which reverses rapidly developing allergic reactions) and barked for an ambulance to be called ASAP. Danny survived, even though he was in critical care for a week and came close to dying. The doctor's position within the company did not survive.

Danny doesn't have much faith in doctors since that episode. Nor should you. There is much ignorance about this topic. Be informed, stay alert and protect yourself or your child. Always challenge the prescribing medic where you suspect he or she is not taking this issue seriously.

It isn't rocket science. It's more important than rocket science. It could be you or your child who suffers needlessly.

IF YOU HAVE EVER HAD A SERIOUS REACTION TO ASPIRIN/ DISPIRIN OR ANY DRUG IN THE NSAID GROUP YOU SHOULD WEAR A MEDIC-ALERT BRACELET AT ALL TIMES TO WARN DOCTORS.

NEVER LET A DOCTOR IGNORE THIS SENSITIVITY. THE INAPPROPRIATE INJECTION OR PRESCRIPTION OF AN NSAID COULD PROVOKE A SEVERE AND LIFE-THREATENING ASTHMATIC ATTACK.

5

Fungal sinusitis

For many years sinus specialists believed that fungal sinus infections only affected a small group of people whose immunity was already compromised. This group included those with HIV or Hepatitis C and people on chemotherapy drugs, which deplete normal immune cells. A significantly compromised immunity cannot fight what are known as 'opportunistic' infections, such as those driven by fungal spores.

However, in recent years there has been a major rethink on this: ear, nose and throat specialists, especially in the USA, consider fungal infections of the sinuses to be much more common, and not just in people with low immunity. Fungal spores can invade the sinus cavities, settle down and make a nice home for themselves. The sinus lining, especially if it is already swollen and irritable, is an ideal breeding ground for this type of micro-organism.

Danny

We met Danny in the last chapter, where I recounted his tale of a serious reaction to an injected anti-inflammatory compound. He is 46 years old, with a 20-year history of nose polyps, fleshy, benign growths that form in the nose and sinuses (see Chapter 6). He has had four separate operations to remove the polyps but they keep recurring (which, unfortunately, is quite common for people with aggressive polyps). In addition, as you may recall from the previous chapter, Danny has asthma and a life-threatening allergy to aspirin and painkillers called NSAIDs. He also has a range of other symptoms that include total loss of sense of smell and very poor sense of taste. To control his nasal polyps and give himself a decent quality of life, Danny takes a large dose of steroid tablets every day. But while this medication does help (and indeed is life saving), there are significant side-effects that include thinning of the bones, weakening of the muscles and tendons and weight gain.

On 28 January 2008 he presented with a worsening of his polyp symptoms and pressure behind his left eye. When he was examined there were found to be polyps occupying about one-third of the upper space in both his nostrils.

These symptoms suggested his polyps were becoming aggressively active and could cause other and more worrying problems such as eye and brain damage (the polyps can burrow out of the sinuses and into brain tissue). An urgent scan was arranged, as well as an urgent appointment with a specialist surgeon. Coincidentally Danny was pre-scribed a special antifungal tablet for a proven fungal toenail infection.

Two weeks later Danny was reviewed. He didn't go for the scan or specialist opinion as his polyp symptoms had settled dramatically, with recovery of his lost sense of smell and enhanced sense of taste. In add-ition his asthma had improved. Danny was sleeping better as well. When examined the polyp tissue had shrivelled back to less than five per cent of its original size.

As well as being an unusual but fascinating insight into one of the most baffling and frustrating nose and sinus problems – nasal polyps – in Danny's case there seems no doubt that his difficul-ties relate to a fungal infection of the sinus tissue. This in turn caused the linings to swell so aggressively that polyps formed. The antifungal tablet, prescribed for a completely separate issue (his fungal toenail infection), caused his nose polyps to shrink dramatically.

Types of fungal sinusitis

The next section is written to try and help you better under-stand fungal sinusitis. It is quite technical and you can skip it if you wish. If you do skip ahead, start again with the section on 'Mould and Chronic Sinusitis' (page 43). Also, since this is not a textbook I can only skim the surface of this affliction, espe-cially as there is no real consensus among specialists as to how common it is and what might be the ideal management.

Fungi are plant-like organisms that lack chlorophyll (a green pigment found in plants and algae. It is vital for photosynthesis, where plants obtain energy from light). Since fungi do not have chlorophyll they must absorb food from dead organic matter. Fungi share with bacteria the important ability to break down complex organic substances of almost every type, and are essential to the recycling of carbon and other elements in the cycle of life. Fungi are supposed to 'eat' only dead things, but sometimes they start gorging when the organism is still alive.

In the past 30 years, there has been a significant increase in the number of recorded fungal infections. This can be attributed to increased public awareness, prescribed therapies to suppress immunity (such as cyclosporine, which 'fools' the body's immune system to prevent organ rejection) and overuse of antibiotics.

When the body's immune system is suppressed, fungi find an opportunity to invade tissue, and a number of side-effects occur. Because these organisms do not require light for food production, they can live in a damp and dark environment. The sinuses, consisting of moist, dark cavities, are a natural home to the invading fungi: hence the phrase 'fungal sinusitis'.

There are four types of fungal sinusitis:

- *Mycetoma fungal sinusitis (MFS)* produces clumps of spores, or a 'fungal ball', within a sinus cavity, most frequently the maxillary sinuses. People susceptible to this infection usually have an effective immune system, but may have experienced trauma or injury to the affected sinus. Generally, the fungus does not cause significant problems apart from a mild sinus discomfort. The non-aggressive nature of this disorder requires a treatment consisting of a simple surgical 'cleaning' of the infected sinus. Antifungal therapy is generally not prescribed.
- *Allergic fungal sinusitis (AFS)* is an allergic reaction to environmental fungal spores finely dispersed in the air. This condition can occur in people with a normal immune system.

They usually have a history of allergic rhinitis (nasal allergy). Thick fungal debris and a carbohydrate-rich secretion called mucin develop in the sinus cavities and must be surgically removed for recovery. Recurrence does sometimes occur, even after a thorough surgical clearance.

- *Chronic indolent sinusitis (CIS)* is an invasive form of fungal sinusitis in people without an identifiable immune deficiency. This form is most commonly found in the Sudan and northern India. The disease progresses over months or years, with features including persisting headaches and a progressive facial swelling that can interfere with sight. Anyone with a compromised immune system can be at risk of this type of sinusitis.

- *Fulminant sinusitis (FS)* is usually seen in people whose immunity is significantly compromised, either because of disease such as HIV or through drugs used to treat malignancies. Fulminant sinusitis leads to progressive destruction of the sinuses and can invade the bony cavities containing the eyeball and brain.

The recommended therapy for both chronic indolent sinusitis and fulminant sinusitis is aggressive surgical removal of the fungal material combined with intravenous antifungal therapy.

Mould and chronic sinusitis

In September 1999, the Mayo Clinic in the USA published results of a study on sinusitis. This demonstrated that 93 per cent of all chronic, or persistent, sinusitis is allergic fungal sinusitis. Simply put, AFS is a delayed allergic-type reaction to mould. Mould is a fungus and the primary culprit of fungal sinusitis. Without proper treatment, the condition becomes persistent.

Even with proper treatment, chronic sinusitis will still persist if exposed mould is not removed as far as is practical. Mould thrives all around us. By identifying the relationship between mould and sinusitis, a doctor will be able to develop a treatment plan that will successfully address the cause, symptoms and condition.

How fungal sinusitis develops

1 You breathe airborne particles containing mould that cause an allergic reaction.
2 This reaction causes small pits to form in the lining of the sinuses.
3 These pits trap mucus so that it cannot drain.
4 The stagnant mucus gets infected. This causes nasal polyps and thickening of the lining of the sinuses, which obstructs the outflow of mucus.
5 The polyps cause more infection.
6 The infection causes more polyps.
7 This causes a vicious cycle that is self-perpetuating.

How can I find out if my sinusitis is due to a mould?

CT scans, blood tests and allergy tests help your treating doctor decide whether your sinusitis is due to a fungal infection. Ideally an aspirate (a sample of tissue from the inside of the sinus) is examined under a microscope to see if mould spores can be identified. However, this is not an easy process to perform and may not be offered routinely by your doctor. Sometimes the diagnosis is based on eliminating all other causes and then working on the assumption that the sinusitis is driven by a fungal infection. A speculative course of treatment may be offered to see if this makes any difference. Because all antifungal medications can create troublesome side-effects with long-term use, your treating specialist will monitor progress with blood tests, CT scans and fibre-optic imagery.

What do I do if my sinusitis is due to a fungal infection?

The golden rule is first to get rid of mould in the air you breathe and second, to get rid of the mould in your nose. This allows blocked sinuses to drain, resulting in long-term relief.

Getting rid of mould in the air you breathe

Moulds can be found in a variety of locations within your home, from the surface of foods to indoor plants and household materials like plywood, drywall or fabric. Moulds are simple, microscopic organisms that need the right temperatures, nutrients and moisture to grow.

Controlling moisture is the key to preventing mould growth. When present in large quantities, mould can cause health problems, including allergic reactions, asthma episodes and respiratory problems. In addition, homeowners can incur large bills for structural damage caused by water or water vapour trapped behind the walls. This is a prime location for the growth of mould. That is why it is important to identify potential situations where mould can grow.

When damage has occurred, take steps to clean and thoroughly dry the area. Remedying the source of the moisture problem is a vital step or, most likely, the mould will grow back.

Preventing mould growth

There are a number of steps you can take to prevent the growh of mould in your home:

- Clean, disinfect and dry surfaces.
- Check for leaks; if these are found, repair and clean any moisture damage caused by the leak.
- Reduce moisture in the home by using ventilation at the source of any moisture. When showering or washing dishes, use an exhaust fan or open a window.

- For good overall moisture control throughout the home, use low speed continuous ventilation, such as a centrally run mechanical ventilation system installed by a qualified contractor.
- Keep relative humidity in your home to between 40 and 50 per cent all year round. This may require a dehumidifier during seasons when air conditioning is in use.
- Vent to the outside clothes dryers, stoves and other appliances that produce moisture.
- Fix all leaks, increase air movement and ventilation, and keep appliance drip pans clean.
- Firewood should be stored outside because it is a source of moisture, fungi and bugs.
- It is a good precaution to always wear gloves, goggles and high quality respiratory protection when cleaning areas affected by mould growth and when removing damaged materials.

Identifying mould

Detecting mould growth is fairly easy. Look for the following:

- visible mould growth (discoloration ranging from white to orange and from green to brown or black);
- musty odours;
- discoloration of building materials in areas where previous water damage has occurred, such as drywall and plaster or plywood.

To test or not to test

Testing for mould is not necessary if you see mould or smell a musty odour. Fixing the moisture problem and following these next steps to remedy the situation is usually the best practice.

Removing mould growth

Once you have identified mould growth in your home, follow these steps to remedy the situation:

- Identify and correct the moisture source (e.g. a leaky roof or window).
- Clean and dry the wet area. (It should be cleaned quickly; mould will grow within 24 to 48 hours.)
- Scrub off the mould with detergent and water.
- Let cleaned areas dry thoroughly overnight.
- Remove or clean any materials affected by the mould.
- Porous materials that have been damaged by mould, such as sheetrock, carpeting and plywood, need to be removed.
- Bag and discard the materials at the work area rather than run the risk of spreading contaminants throughout the home.
- Provide continuous and controlled ventilation in the work area, with the area of contamination kept at a negative pressure in relationship to the rest of the home. (In other words, air should flow from clean to dirty areas.)

Avoiding future problems

Once you have removed the mould growth and fixed the source of the problem, make sure you and your home do not sustain further damage by checking regularly for the following symptoms:

- condensation on windows
- cracking or staining of plasterboard
- loosening of drywall tape
- warping wood
- musty odours

Treating the effects of mould in your nose

In addition, you should take the following steps to get rid of mould in your nose, and to counteract its effects:

- Irrigate your nose with Neilmed Sinus Rinse at least twice a day. This washes the mould and other particles out of the nose. There's more on this technique (called nasal douching) in Chapter 12.

- Use a facial steamer when infected or congested to breathe steam into the nose.
- Take any prescribed medications. This may involve oral antibiotics, oral antifungal compounds or antifungal nose sprays. Antifungal nose sprays are more commonly used in the USA than elsewhere so it may not be easy to get hold of them. However, if your treating specialist believes you would benefit from them, he'll know how to get the products to you.
- You may need sinus surgery to clear any obstructed sinus openings.
- Steroid nose sprays and tablets are often used to reduce the unpleasant side-effects of this condition.
- If your doctor recommends immunotherapy as part of your treatment (see Chapter 10), then go for it.
- Take immune boosters such as thymus vitamins.

Summary

Fungal sinusitis exists. The problem for anyone with stubborn sinusitis is how to find out whether or not his or her condition is fungal related. The tests and investigations are not foolproof. The treatments are also not agreed. What might be suggested in London could be completely different to what is prescribed in Paris, and there are even regional variations of opinion throughout the USA. Be aware of the condition. Equally, be aware of the limitations of investigations and treatments. Danny's success story is a rare event. And he's still being monitored to see if his condition fully settles with oral antifungal tablets.

6

Nose polyps

Nose polyps are soft, grape-like growths that spread out from the sinuses or form on the surface of the nasal lining. They are the end result of many different irritations within the nose and sinuses, from allergy to fungal and/or bacterial infection; often the cause cannot be identified. Most polyps start near the ethmoid sinuses (located at the top of the inside of the nose) and grow into the open areas. They are usually visible inside the nose. Indeed, if you'd like to see some digital images of nasal polyps, check out

<http://www.allergy-ireland.ie/dedicated_sinusitis_facility.php>.

When polyps develop the nose becomes blocked, creating breathing difficulties. Polyps also obstruct the sinus cavities, creating stagnant secretions that are an ideal breeding ground for microorganisms such as bacteria and fungi. And when sinuses become

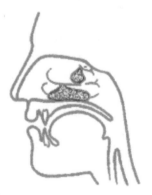

Figure 6.1 Nasal polyps

infected as a result of these secretions, it causes sinusitis (inflammation of the sinus cavities), with all the symptoms I have already described:

- nasal obstruction
- a runny nose
- recurring sinus infections
- dull headaches
- snoring
- persistent stuffiness
- difficulty in breathing
- post-nasal drip
- thick, discoloured nasal drainage
- reduced sense of smell and taste
- facial pain

Charles

Forty-nine-year-old Charles is in great distress. He walks the floor at night unable to rest. Within 30 minutes or so of falling asleep he wakens, gasping for air. He's started to wheeze during the daytime and gets breathless with even slight exertion. He's been checked carefully in case this is the first sign of heart failure but his cardiac status is normal. A presumptive diagnosis of late-onset asthma is made and appropriate anti-asthma medicine prescribed. This helps his daytime symptoms but not his night-time misery. All blood tests are normal, his chest X-ray clear. Allergy testing is negative.

Further questioning reveals that he snores heavily, has a very poor sense of smell and a possibly reduced sense of taste. His wife gives a detailed history of his convulsive gasps of breathing during the night and has taken to sleeping in the spare room. A diagnosis of sleep apnoea (see Chapter 9) is now considered.

Fibre-optic assessment of his nose and sinuses shows a severely swollen nose lining with aggressive fluid 'blistering', causing polyps to form.

Charles responds to medical therapy (as explained later in this chapter). He has his best night's sleep for quite some time and can smell again.

What causes polyps to form?

I wish I knew. I can tell you of several theories but, in truth, some types of nose polyps defy medical understanding. Several interrelating factors are thought to combine to produce inflammation of the nose and sinus linings. This causes the tissues to swell and form the grape-like growths. When a bright light is directed at the tissue it has the look of small boggy, damp sacs (doctors use the word *oedema* to describe such changes). These bags of fluid can enlarge and pop out through the sinus openings and into the nasal cavity. The bulging tissue is now termed a *nose polyp*.

Possible trigger factors include:

- Continuous inflammation within the nose and sinuses. This is the main cause of nasal polyps. This inflammation can be related to allergy, atmospheric pollution or even an aggressive (or recurring) sinus infection.
- Overproduction of fluid in the nose and sinus linings, causing a blistering-type phenomenon. The normally shiny pink membranes change to a dull grey colour.

Who is at risk of getting nasal polyps?

- Polyps are more common in adults older than 40, and children with conditions such as asthma, chronic sinus infections (sinusitis), dust mite and pollen allergy (allergic sinusitis) and cystic fibrosis (an inherited disorder that causes respiratory disease).
- There is a 1 to 20 in 1,000 chance of a normal person developing nasal polyps (this declines after the age of 60).
- The occurrence in the normal population is 0.1 per cent in children and about 1 per cent in adults.
- There is a gender difference – two to four males to every female will develop polyps.

- There is no racial variation (it doesn't matter whether you're European, Asian or African, the same statistics apply).

How do I get rid of my nose polyps?

There are only two options for treatment: medical or surgical. *Medical* treatment means that specific prescribed drugs are used, first to shrink the polyp tissue back as far as possible and then to stabilize the area with special nose sprays. It's very like the treatment plan I explained in Chapter 3 and I'll run a typical strategy again below. *Surgical* treatment means what it says on the tin: the polyps are cut out using a procedure called polypectomy or functional endoscopic sinus surgery (both explained later in this chapter).

Medical treatment for nose polyps

Nose polyps can be shrunk using the same Betnesol steroid drops I described in Chapter 3. Figure 3.2 on page 22 shows how the drops are used. You lie on a couch or bed so that your head can bend to a 90-degree angle, either forwards or backwards. The idea is to allow the prescribed drops to trickle around the polyps, coat all the tissue and find a resting point at the 'ceiling' level of the nose. The medicine slowly shrinks the polyp tissue. How long the drops are used depends on how big the polyps are at the start of treatment. Typically therapy can last for weeks, even a month.

When the polyps are sufficiently shrunk, a steroid nose spray is used to stabilize the nasal cavity and prevent the polyp tissue re-forming. The spray (and there are a number of excellent products – Nasacort, Flixonase, Avamys or Nasonex – See Chapter 3) is directed into the now normal-looking nose in a dosage decided by the doctor treating you. The purpose is to maintain the improvement achieved by the Betnesol drops. If you just treat with drops and stop as soon as normality is achieved, unfortunately the polyps will re-form. So it's very important not only to shrink the polyps but then keep them shrunk. Here's a typical regime for an adult.

Using Betnesol nose drops for nasal polyps

- Get into the position suggested (see Figure 3.2 on p. 22).
- Instil two drops into each nostril (it might be easier to have someone help you with this as it's not easy to concentrate on the correct position *and* ensure you're getting the drops in properly).
- Stay in the position for three minutes.
- After the three minutes pinch the soft part of your nose closed. Now lift your head to the normal position (some drops may spill out at this point but that's not important).
- Do this three times daily for 30 days.
- On day 31 start the nasal spray. The dosage is two squiffs up into each nostril (as shown in Figure 3.2) twice daily.

For some people with nose polyps, oral anti-allergy medicines (see Chapter 3) such as Singulair or Accolate may be added. These can prove very effective in controlling nose polyps and preventing regrowth. While they are strictly anti-allergy compounds, they may work where no allergic trigger can be identified.

Quite often the polyps can be so large and 'established' inside the nose that the Betnesol drops won't penetrate the tissue. Here a high dose of steroid tablets works wonders. However, because oral steroids cause considerable side-effects, this strategy is not used often and then only in selected cases. The steroid tablets are called Deltacortril and their strength is 5 milligrams.

Because they can damage the stomach when used in high doses a special compound called Omeprazole is also taken. Omeprazole protects the stomach lining during the steroid treatment. With this strategy the high dose of steroids shrinks the nose polyps to a level where treatment nose sprays can penetrate the nasal cavity and exert their anti-polyp effect. Table 6.1 shows a typical treatment regime. Here I have combined the oral steroids with steroid drops (Betnesol) for a quicker and (hopefully) more sustained result. However, this must only be considered in consultation with your treating doctor.

After shrinking the polyps, your doctor may prescribe medication to control any associated allergies or infection. These include antihistamines, leukotriene receptor antagonists (as mentioned in Chapter 3) or an antibiotic if there is the hint of

Table 6.1 Shrinking nose polyps

Days	Steroid tablets	Additional treatments
1–5	Deltacortril 5 mg: take eight all together half an hour after breakfast	Betnesol nose drops: two twice daily into each nostril Singulair 10 mg (one tablet) at night. Start on day 1 and continue until a decision is made on its effectiveness Neilmed Sinus Rinse (see Chapter 12) twice daily to clear the nose of mucus and debris once the polyps have shrunk Omeprazole 40 mg, one each day for 20 days
6–10	Deltacortril 5 mg: take six all together half an hour after breakfast	Betnesol nose drops: two twice daily into each nostril Neilmed Sinus Rinse twice daily Omeprazole 40 mg, one each day
11–15	Deltacortril 5 mg: take four all together half an hour after breakfast	On day 15 start the steroid nose spray (Avamys, Nasacort, Nasonex or Flixonase): three squiffs into each nostril twice daily, continuing until review Neilmed Sinus Rinse twice daily Omeprazole 40 mg, one each day
16–20	Deltacortril 5 mg: take two together half an hour after breakfast	Neilmed Sinus Rinse twice daily Omeprazole 40 mg, one each day

a background sinus infection. Antifungal medications may also be considered (see previous chapter). Some cases of nose polyps may be triggered by an unusual immune system response to a fungus (this, for example, was the explanation for Danny's situation in Chapter 5). Surgical removal of fungal debris will almost always be necessary.

Surgical removal of nose polyps

When all medical therapies fail either to shrink your nose polyps, or successfully to stop them re-forming, then a surgical option is your only chance for a better quality of life. The type of operation depends on the size, number and location of the polyps. Options for nasal polyp surgery include:

- *Polypectomy.* Small or isolated polyps can often be completely removed using a small mechanical suction device or a micro-debrider (an instrument that cuts and extracts soft tissue). The procedure, called a polypectomy, is performed on an outpatient basis. After polypectomy, you'll be treated for any underlying inflammation, usually with steroid nasal drops and sprays and sometimes with antibiotics or oral steroids. Even so, polyps may recur and you may need surgery more than once.
- *Functional endoscopic sinus surgery.* This is a more extensive procedure that not only removes polyps, but also opens the part of the sinus cavity where polyps usually form. If your sinuses are very blocked or inflamed, your doctor may deliberately widen the opening into the sinus cavities.

In both cases, the surgeon uses a thin, rigid tube and a camera called a video endoscope. Because endoscopic surgery requires small incisions, you generally heal more quickly and with less discomfort than with other types of surgery. Still, full recovery may take several weeks.

Nose polyps and their link with asthma

Throughout this book I have written about the link between sinusitis and asthma. Just to refresh your memory:

- Sinusitis involves the nose as well as the sinuses.
- Sinusitis may cause nose and sinus symptoms only.
- Sinusitis may provoke chest symptoms as well.
- Sinusitis may coexist with asthma.

Well, you can replace sinusitis with nose polyps in the above and the same principles apply. Nose polyps may be confined to the nose and sinuses and cause symptoms only there, *or* they may coexist with asthma. When there is asthma with nose polyps the asthma tends to be aggressive, so it is important to keep the nose polyps under control. If the nose polyps become infected or become so large they irritate the nose and sinuses, then it's likely that they will aggravate any background asthma.

Nose polyps, asthma and aspirin allergy

There is a very important condition called Samter's triad (yet another medical term), where three difficult problems coexist in the same person: nose polyps, asthma and an exquisite sensitivity or allergy to aspirin. Here are some basic facts about this condition:

- It starts typically in the third and fourth decades of life.
- It is more common in females and in otherwise non-allergic individuals.
- Ingestion of aspirin or an NSAID (see Chapter 4) induces a dangerous reaction within minutes.
- Symptoms include facial flushing, perspiration and intense lethargy, streaming nose, nasal congestion, conjunctivitis and wheezing. Some individuals develop abdominal symptoms such as cramping and diarrhoea. A severe reaction can kill.
- Surgery for nose polyps is usually less successful in aspirin-

sensitive people compared with aspirin-tolerant individuals, with polyp formation quite common and frequent.

• Aspirin desensitization can be carried out in a hospital setting. This involves giving small doses of aspirin over a long period of time with a view to tricking the person's immunity into finally accepting aspirin and not triggering severe reactions if exposed. This is a hazardous strategy and must only be carried out by experienced doctors and in a hospital where back-up support is available.

While it may seem simple to advise a person so affected to avoid aspirin, the issue is more complicated. *The presence of aspirin is not always obvious.* It is present in many across-the-counter painkillers as well as various sinus tablets, medicines used to control period pain, and cold and flu tablets. If you are sensitive to aspirin, you will need to read medicine labels carefully and be cautious about taking any analgesic without talking to your doctor or pharmacist first. *You will even have to be careful of some foods, and very careful that your doctor does not prescribe you any medication which may contain aspirin.* I've stated how this applies more fully in Chapter 4. The same principles apply here. I *strongly* recommend you now turn back to page 33 and carefully read through the information on exactly where aspirin – and its chemical component sodium salicylate – occurs. As already stated there, it's better to learn these facts reading this book than to hear about them in the intensive care unit of your local hospital. And remember:

NEVER LET A DOCTOR IGNORE THIS SENSITIVITY. THE INAPPROPRIATE INJECTION OR PRESCRIPTION OF AN NSAID COULD PROVOKE A SEVERE AND LIFE-THREATENING ASTHMATIC ATTACK.

7

The sinusitis epidemic

The number of people, especially children, troubled with sinusitis has increased over the last decade. In the UK and Ireland there are approximately 8.5 million people with sinusitis spending millions of pounds and euros on sinus relief products. In the USA, health experts estimate that 37 million Americans are affected by sinusitis every year. Healthcare providers report nearly 32 million cases of chronic sinusitis to the Centres for Disease Control and Prevention annually. Americans spend $5.8 billion each year on healthcare costs related to sinusitis.

While there are many different causes of sinusitis, this increase particularly reflects the surge in allergy-related conditions. It is also putting an extra burden on already overstretched health services.

Unfortunately in the UK and Ireland there aren't enough facilities to deal with the demand for allergy investigation. In Britain this was investigated by a House of Commons committee, and their findings make for depressing reading. In short the Committee found a 'serious epidemic' of allergy and the Department of Health agreed. Allergy care in the NHS was totally inadequate at all levels, with a postcode lottery of premium care. In Ireland it's no better, indeed it's maybe even worse.

The following statistics highlight the problem:

- Eighteen million people in Britain (out of a population of 60 million) have some type of allergy.
- Three million will need to see a specialist in allergy because of multi-organ involvement (in other words, allergy affecting

more than one area: eyes, nose, chest, skin, etc.) or because of the complexity of the condition.

- Children are particularly affected. Over 40,000 of the children born each year will develop allergy.
- One in 50 children have a nut allergy, apart from other food allergies.
- Allergy has become more complex and severe. At least 10 per cent of children and young adults with allergy have more than one allergic disorder.
- The NHS has six full-time specialist allergy centres – and less than 30 consultant allergy doctors. Many of these doctors are employed in research and so their time for clinical work is restricted. Some parts of the country have no specialist allergists, and family doctors in these areas have no one to turn to for practical advice.

So what happens to people with allergy when they need specialist help? Quite often it turns out to be a frustrating experience. Consider this typical runaround of a boy with troublesome atopic (allergic) eczema. His main problem is his skin and that's what motivates his parents to seek expert attention. While they are with the dermatologist (skin doctor) they might mention that the boy is 'chesty' (*asthma*). 'That's not my area,' they're told, 'you must bring him to a chest doctor.' At the chest doctor they wonder about the boy's constant blocked nose and repeated head colds (*sinusitis*). 'That's not my problem,' trumpets the chest doctor, 'you must bring him to an ear, nose and throat doctor.' At the ENT division they mention the boy rubs at his eyes a lot and the whites are very red (*conjunctivitis*). 'Take him to an eye doctor,' they are advised.

Why an ear, nose and throat doctor won't look at the eyes as part of his work for the nasal problem escapes logic. Why the chest physician refuses to inspect the nasal cavity when assessing the possible asthma symptoms is also illogical.

This inter-department referral is disillusioning for children and parents. It suggests a lack of understanding of the background problem. Could this boy really have so many different conditions, or is he suffering an allergic challenge to the various systems, eyes, nose, chest, etc.? You don't have to be Einstein to make the connection, yet it is often denied. It seems easier to ignore and keep referring than to look at the bigger picture and determine a structured management strategy.

- Many dermatologists refuse to accept an allergic link in atopic eczema even though it's screaming for attention.
- Many paediatricians refuse to do allergy tests, even where there is an overwhelming allergic link to presenting symptoms. ('Lift the carpets ... get rid of the dog ... try stopping milk' – these are some of the many snippets of advice I've heard. Much money is spent on anti-dust mite manoeuvres when the child doesn't have a dust mite allergy.)
- Expensive and inappropriate anti-asthma drugs are prescribed without any reference to the background allergic cause.

Perhaps the most baffling aspect is the indifference shown at all levels of the health system. With statistics suggesting that so many of the population have some type of allergy, there are more resources devoted to cardiovascular and osteoporosis screening programmes and suchlike than to providing even a minimal allergy service. It's disappointing to say the least.

Which takes me back to the sinusitis epidemic. It *is* a reflection of the allergy epidemic and this may be caused by a number of factors, possibly inter-reacting with one another. They include:

- *The hygiene hypothesis:* clean living isn't necessarily good for us. By depriving our immune system of key infections caused by viruses, bacteria and parasites, we fail to develop the necessary tolerance for ordinarily tame foreign particles. The immune system – underused and spoiling for a fight – goes overboard when finally given the opportunity, no matter how slight the opponent. Poor people living in developing countries exhibit markedly lower levels of allergy. This holds true even for impoverished communities within polluted urban centres. Dirt, in other words, may be good for you. But poor people living in developing countries can become allergic when they move to a more developed area (see the following case history).

- *Atmospheric pollution:* persistent exposure to particulate matter due to automobile exhaust in urban settings increases the risks of developing allergies and exacerbates asthma. Japan is a classic example of industrialization's downside. In the 1930s, hay fever hadn't yet been recognized. However, from 1970 onwards 15 per cent of Japanese schoolchildren showed signs of hay fever. Perhaps that country's rapid industrialization and pollution swamped the protective immunity of Japanese children?

- *Over-exposure to antibiotics:* over the past 40 years, as widespread antibiotic use has climbed, so too have allergy rates.

Abasiofun

Abasiofun is 24. She lived in Nigeria all her life before moving to Ireland in 2007. At home in rural Nigeria her lifestyle was simple and her accommodation basic. She shared a concrete brick house under a thatched roof with her four siblings and her parents. There were no carpets or curtains and minimal furniture. There were animals in the neighbourhood, cattle and dogs especially, but no domestic pets.

She started working in Ireland in a country house in February 2007. The owners kept horses and went riding daily. They had dogs that more or less had the run of the downstairs living area and cats that sneaked into any room with an open door. Within one month of living and working in this environment, Abasiofun developed severe head colds and sneezing attacks. Her employers consoled her that this was just a response to Ireland's cold and damp conditions, a contrast to the hot and dry Nigerian climate she'd grown up in. Abasiofun grinned and hoped they were right. But she felt miserable. Indeed she'd never felt like this before in her life. Back home she'd been healthy and well, never requiring medical attention.

Abasiofun's head colds got worse and she had difficulty sleeping at night. She was noticeably breathless with exertion. As the weeks went on she became wheezy and her breathing was laboured. Her skin, once smooth and unblemished, was now itchy and irritable. She was scratching at it, something she'd never done before. Not wanting to be a nuisance so early in her employment, she kept her symptoms to herself.

By week 12 of living in the country house, Abasiofun was so unwell she had to visit the local doctor. He recognized that the young woman had a severe sinusitis that was triggering asthma. He also noticed she was developing eczema (itchy skin) in the areas usually seen in children, the creases of the knees and elbows. As part of her check-up, the doctor ordered allergy tests. The results showed that Abasiofun was severely allergic to horsehair, dust mites and cat hair. Minute particles, smaller than a speck of dust, of these allergy-provoking substances had swept inside the girl's nose and sinuses, triggering an aggressive allergic sinusitis. This in turn kickstarted asthma and, slowly but gradually, eczema.

Abasiofun quit the country house. In fact she quit Ireland too, and returned to her native Nigeria and better health.

Abasiofun must have been carrying the genetic code for allergy all her life. However, her basic living conditions and lifestyle in Nigeria did not challenge her immune system and so she stayed well. The move to a damp and colder climate was one shock to her system. An even greater jolt was the high amount of allergy-provoking material she suddenly became exposed to. Her immunity was challenged like never before and Abasiofun started showing all the signs of a highly allergic individual. She first developed sinusitis, then asthma and finally eczema. (In babies such allergic events occur in the reverse order: i.e. eczema, followed by nose and sinus allergy and eventually asthma.)

When I spoke with Abasiofun I asked her what was the worst feature of her ill-health. 'The sinus pains, doctor,' she replied, sniffing and snorting, hands full of damp tissues. 'Please make my sinuses better.'

I did. But she still went back to Nigeria.

For most sinus patients, moving to a drier, warmer, low-allergy climate isn't an option. But if Abasiofun's story highlights anything (and graphically too), having sinusitis makes you feel absolutely miserable.

8

How sinusitis affects children: allergic irritability syndrome

Sinus problems make people feel quite miserable – these's no argument there. However, sinus problems in children, if unrecognized or badly managed, can have a significant toll on their emotional as well as physical well-being.

For years I've been dealing with children troubled by multiple allergy problems and I've wondered how they get through a full school day. What with their itchy eczematous skin, their snuffly and irritable noses and wheezy chests, they carry a significant burden of ill-health. Adults know how to complain (and rarely hold back), whereas some children don't know any better. They think everyone goes around with a bunged-up nose, wheezy chest and an almost perpetual tiredness. If the sinusitis is aggressive the child may get intermittent hearing loss. So one day he's bright and alert in class, interreacting and cooperating. Next day he seems distant and detached, ignoring questions or not fully grasping what's going on. The teachers are at a loss to explain these variations in attentiveness and the boy's parents can't quite understand the situation either. It's not uncommon for these children to be labelled 'difficult'.

Sinusitis also provokes intense fatigue. If an affected child is not treated he misses out on ordinary children's activities and can be isolated and ignored. He's not picked for the football team even though he loves the game. And if he's picked he's usually last choice and then put in goal, out of harm's way. Secretly he'd love to be a striker, fast-footed and skilful. He knows he's well able to take the ball around defences. If only he could get the chance. If only he didn't feel so tired all the time. If only he didn't have to stop every five yards to blow his nose, if only he didn't have to take a puff of his asthma inhaler in front of everyone. If only, if only ...

I've been talking about this for years to the point of being considered a crank. Then an article appeared in a reputable medical journal that summarized my observations to a tee.[1] Suddenly I knew how right I'd been. Now I realized that I wasn't the only one making these comments. The difference was that while my observations were no more than just that, observations, the authors of this piece had the scientific background to stand over their claims.

The term *allergic irritability syndrome* has been coined to explain the many unpleasant symptoms and features children with untreated allergic rhino-sinusitis may show. Allergic rhino-sinusitis (ARS) is a fancy medical term for allergy-driven nose and sinus problems.

So here goes. Here are some of the effects children with unrecognized (and therefore untreated) ARS may experience:

- a significantly impaired quality of life;
- significant learning difficulties;
- a lower ability to achieve different types of knowledge (factual, conceptual and knowledge application) compared with healthy children;
- sleep apnoea (more on this in Chapter 9), snoring and disturbed sleep patterns, in turn leading to daytime drowsiness, grumpy mood and poor school performance;
- impaired hearing, if fluid collects in the inner ear (the medical term for this is *serous otitis media*);
- repeated 'head colds' that go down to the chest (which is

[1] H. P. van Bever and P. C. Potter, 'Making the allergic child happy: treating more than symptoms', *Clinical & Experimental Allergy Reviews*, 6, 6–9.

really an untreated nose and sinus allergy triggering early asthma);

- nasal blockage and irritation (sneezing, rubbing at the nose to relieve the itch);
- dark circles around the eyes with puffiness of the lower lids;
- poor concentration, disruptive behaviour and unexplained mood swings.

In severe cases it may also cause or at least contribute to attention deficit hyper-activity disorder (ADHD).

I recall one six-year-old boy who told his parents that he felt angry all the time when unwell with his allergic sinusitis. This is sad and unnecessary as allergic sinusitis is easily managed, especially in children. The treatment strategies outlined in Chapter 3 apply to adults and children.

Almost all sinus problems begin inside the nose.

Effects of sinusitis in children

Set out below in more detail are the common effects of persisting sinusitis in children.

Nasal congestion

Allergies are the most common cause of chronic nasal congestion in children. Sometimes a child's nose is congested (obstructed) to the point that he or she breathes through the mouth, especially while sleeping.

If the congestion is left untreated this forces air currents through the mouth. The strength of the air changes the way the soft bones of the face grow. The features may become abnormally elongated in a pattern called 'adenoidal face'. This causes the teeth to come in at an improper angle as well as creating an overbite. Braces or other dental treatments may be necessary to correct these problems.

Allergy and ear infections

Allergies lead to inflammation in the ear and may cause fluid accumulation, triggering ear infections and decreased hearing. If this happens when the child is learning to talk, poor speech development may result. Allergies can also cause earaches and ear itching, popping and fullness ('stuffed-up ears').

Allergies at school

Autumn is back to school time. For allergic children that may mean absences due to allergy flare-ups. The following are some of the problems to look for so that the condition can be properly diagnosed and treated, as well as several suggestions for helping the allergic child:

- *Dust irritation*. Reducing dust in the home will be helpful to most allergic family members. At school, children with allergy problems should sit away from the blackboard to avoid irritation from chalk dust.
- *School pets*. Furry animals in school may cause problems for allergic children. If your child has more problems while at school, it could be the class pet.
- *Asthma and physical education*. Sports are a big part of the school day. Having asthma does not mean eliminating these activities. Often medication administered by using an inhaler is prescribed before exercise to control the symptoms. A child with asthma and other allergic diseases should be able to participate in any sport the child chooses – provided the doctor's advice is followed.
- *Dry air*. With the onset of cold weather, using a humidifier to accompany forced air heating systems may be helpful in some regions of the country. Adding a small amount of moisture to dry air makes breathing easier for most people. However, care should be taken not to allow the humidity above 40 per cent, which promotes the growth of dust mites and mould.

● *Change in behaviour.* Children cannot always vocalize their annoying or painful symptoms. Their discomfort may manifest as behaviour problems. Be on the alert for possible allergies if your child has bouts of irritability, temper tantrums or decreased ability to concentrate in school. These may be signs of allergic irritability syndrome. Sometimes allergic children are badly behaved and have short attention spans. Needless to say their school work suffers. When a child's allergies are properly treated, his or her symptoms, behaviour and school performance can improve dramatically.

Jack

Jack, aged eight, is a problematic child at home and at school. He seems constantly agitated, ill at ease with himself and disruptive. His teachers complain that he's troublesome, irritable, cranky and hard to handle. When they mention this to his parents they hear their own concerns echoed by Jack's mum and dad. They too find the boy difficult.

In case there's a physical cause for his behaviour Jack is brought to the family doctor for a check-up. Within the first few minutes of the consultation the doctor notices how much Jack is agitated by his nose. He's constantly rubbing at it, dragging his sleeve along the nostril openings, snorting and snuffling. When the doctor inspects the inside lining of Jack's nose he realizes immediately that the boy has an aggressive nose and sinus allergy. He arranges for a battery of tests, including an allergy screen. Surprisingly the only abnormal reaction to show up is that Jack has a strong horsehair allergy. 'That makes no sense,' complain both parents. 'We're miles away from any horses and Jack doesn't even like going near them.' But the family doctor, wise man that he is, recognizes that something has to be irritating Jack's nose and sinuses. He advises the boy's parents to check their house carefully for horsehair.

Two days later he gets a delighted telephone call. Jack sleeps in a room on his own. But there is a spare bed in that room for the occasional visitor. The bed was inherited from an elderly uncle and the mattress is stuffed with horsehair. Jack uses the bed as a trampoline. Every time he jumps up and down on it he disturbs the horsehair. This enters his nose and sinuses, which in turn causes havoc with their delicate membranes. And this is the background allergic challenge to Jack's ill-health.

Out go the horsehair bed and mattress. Jack's room is steam cleaned to remove any residual traces of horsehair. Then his troublesome allergic sinusitis is successfully treated with medicine.

The boy improves dramatically. His mood, personality, temperament and behaviour recover to normal limits within a week. Jack's parents are astonished. Jack's teachers are delighted. Jack's doctor is pleased as Punch at his diagnostic skills. And Jack is a much more contented child. Jack has been suffering from allergic irritability syndrome.

However, not every doctor has the insight to check for this condition and the skill to know how to manage it correctly. There are a lot of unhappy Jacks in the world who don't know what it's like to have a normally functioning and not-irritated nose and sinuses.

Allergic diseases and cognitive impairment

Sneezing, wheezing, watery eyes and a runny nose aren't the only symptoms of allergic diseases. Many people with allergic sinusitis also report feeling 'slower' and drowsy. When their allergies act up they have trouble concentrating and remembering.

For instance, nose and sinus allergy can be associated with:

- decreased ability to concentrate and function
- activity limitation
- decreased decision-making capacity
- impaired hand-eye coordination
- problems remembering things
- irritability
- sleep disorders
- fatigue
- missed days at work or school
- school injuries

Causes

Experts believe the main factors contributing to cognitive impairment in people with allergic sinusitis are sleep interruption and over-the-counter (OTC) medications.

Secondary factors, such as blockage of the Eustachian tube

(ear canal), can cause hearing problems, with a negative impact on learning and comprehension. Constant nose blowing and coughing can interrupt concentration and the learning process, and allergy-related absences can cause people to miss school or work and subsequently fall behind.

Sleep disruption

Chronic (ongoing) nasal congestion can cause difficulty in breathing, especially at night. If your child has a significant nose and sinus allergy he or she may awaken a dozen times a night. Falling asleep again can be difficult, cutting short the total number of sleep hours. Losing just a few hours of sleep can lead to a significant decrease in your child's ability to function. Prolonged loss of sleep can cause difficulty in concentration, inability to remember things, and can contribute to accidents. Night after night of interrupted sleep can cause serious decreases in learning ability and performance in school.

Over-the-counter medications

Many over-the-counter sinus therapies (especially antihistamines) adversely affect mental functioning. Indeed some allergy therapies may even cause cognitive or mental impairment.

Children often cannot speak for themselves when trying to explain their sense of ill-health. Persisting sinusitis, be it allergic or not, can trigger often dramatic problems for children. With allergic disorders on the rise worldwide (as we saw in Chapter 7), the plight of the untreated allergic child is not a happy one. However, with correct identification and treatments this should not be an ongoing problem for any child.

9

How sinusitis can affect sleep and trigger skin problems

Sleep apnoea

Simple medical problems can surface in strange ways. In the USA police confronted the parents of a seven-year-old boy and questioned them about physical abuse. The next-door neighbour had reported that the child was awake regularly during the night and screaming in a state of terror. The parents admitted this but couldn't explain the situation. They denied abuse, physical or otherwise. A local doctor checked the boy and found no sign of abuse but significant breathing problems. He couldn't breathe through his nose and his chin was dropped in a reflexive, self-protective manner. The parents claimed he had been like that since infancy but didn't think it unusual.

The boy was admitted to hospital and discovered to have severe sleep apnoea (intermittent and recurring episodes where he stopped breathing). When he was examined under anaesthetic it was found that he had adenoid swelling so large it obstructed his nose completely (the adenoid is spongy tissue located at the back of the throat that can block breathing through the nose). Surgical removal produced a dramatic and instant cure. The boy started to sleep normally and there were no more night terrors. The neighbour was thanked. The police backed off. Order was restored.

A blocked or obstructed nose can cause a multitude of medical problems, some simple and others more problematic. In adults and children the usual cause is an allergic swelling of the nose lining. Children can also get blockage at the back of the throat

70

due to enlarged adenoids. Interference with sleep can become a major issue here. ARS – allergic rhino-sinusitis, or an allergic challenge to the nose and sinuses – may cause sleep apnoea. In plain English this means that the nose is so obstructed that the adult or child cannot breathe through it properly at night. People snore heavily and the pattern of snoring is something like this: *snore, snore, snore, snore, snore, snore, snooooorrrreeee, snoooooorrrrrreeeeee, snooooooorrrrreeeeee* ... no breathing at all ... for quite some time ... *SNORRRRRRRRTTTTTTT, yawn,* slightly normal breathing and then back to *snore, snore, snore,* etc.

The no-breathing episodes can last for 20, 30 or even 40 seconds at a time and this pattern continues through the night. The end result is oxygen-starvation episodes that deprive the snorer (and anyone unfortunate enough to be in the same room!) of restful, restorative sleep. While this might read as amusing, in reality it's a serious health concern. For adults, persisting sleep apnoea can put pressure on the cardiovascular system. Common features include:

- excessive daytime sleepiness, e.g. falling asleep at work, while driving, during conversation or when watching TV
- irritability, short temper
- morning headaches
- forgetfulness
- changes in mood or behaviour
- anxiety or depression
- decreased interest in sex

With children it leads to daytime drowsiness, grumpy mood and poor school performance. In severe cases it may cause or at least contribute to attention deficit hyper-activity disorder.

It is estimated that the number of children with blocked noses, be it due to allergy or swollen adenoids/tonsils, could be as high as 25 per cent. That's a lot of kids with disturbed sleep (among other symptoms). And it means there are a lot of parents out there wondering just what *is* wrong with their child.

Almost all sinus problems begin inside the nose.

Hives (urticaria) in adults and children

If this section seems repetitive then I apologize. However, there's no other way to explain the link between sinusitis and hives (the medical term for which is *urticaria*) than by going back over some of the material from Chapter 3. Do refer back and have a look at the illustration of the nose and the sinuses on page 20 (Figure 3.1).

The lining of the nose is delicate and therefore easily damaged. Running along the inside are three shelf-like structures called *turbinates*. These clean, filter, warm and moisten the air we breathe before it enters the lungs. But the turbinates are easily injured. Ignoring physical trauma, any challenge that aggressively irritates the nasal lining may cause the turbinates to swell. The challenge can range from infection to allergy, from cigarette smoking to inhaling chemical vapours, etc. When the turbinates swell they block the little tubes that drain the sinuses into the nose. Now we not only have a nose problem but the beginning of sinusitis. If the swelling within the nose persists the sinuses cannot breathe, their air pockets stagnate and become a rich feeding ground for infection with viruses, moulds and bacteria. Running along the ceiling of the nose is an exquisitely delicate nerve ending that transmits the sensations of *taste* and *smell* to the brain. With prolonged pressure on this nerve from turbinate swelling these sensations fade.

The first to go is the sense of smell, usually a subtle and gradual loss over some months. Once the sense of smell has almost totally disappeared, the sense of taste becomes impaired. And it is the sense of taste for spice that wilts at the beginning. Now the person with sinus trouble finds most foods taste bland

and goes for spicier products. Unwittingly she now consumes higher amounts of the additives used by the food industry to spice up products. Chief culprit in this group is monosodium glutamate (MSG), also known as E621, a widely used flavouring agent in pre-packed, prepared and take-away foods, especially Chinese, Indian, Thai and similar Oriental cooking.

Jennifer

Jennifer is a 19-year-old student. She did exceptionally well in her final state examinations and now studies law in Dublin. Jennifer also has recurring sinusitis with impaired senses of smell and taste. Jennifer grew up in a small country town on the south coast of Ireland. Before moving to university she lived at home with her parents and had a healthy diet with mainly home-cooked food. But everything home cooked tasted rather bland and Jennifer kept asking for something with a bit of spice in it. Mother refused. She preferred good, wholesome produce, and rarely used tins, packets, bottles or artificial stock cubes when preparing dinner. So Jennifer's wish for spice went unsatisfied.

Once Jennifer left to continue her studies she started to lead her own life, away from the constraints of her parents. She preferred the city night lights to the college library. She wanted experiences far removed from small-town Ireland. And she didn't want to waste time cooking. So she ate out a lot, or bought in, or grabbed fast and easy foods, such as cardboard soups-in-a-cup, cardboard instant rice dishes, cardboard instant curries and pre-cooked spicy chicken wings. The easier the food to prepare, the more attractive it was to Jennifer. And she enjoyed this produce better; she could actually taste something for a change. It at least had a tang to revitalize her jaded palate.

Unwittingly, Jennifer was swallowing a significant number of food additives. The tang in her diet was created by chemicals, mainly monosodium glutamate.

One evening she came out in a very itchy rash, hives as she recognized it. The rash subsided with an antihistamine. Then one evening her upper lip swelled, and the hives returned with a vengeance. It took days and a lot of antihistamines to calm her skin. Finally, one evening after a Chinese meal, Jennifer's lips, face and tongue swelled. Her sinuses became inflamed, painful and congested. The hives returned and this time didn't go away, despite double the usual dosage of antihistamines.

An ingredient in the Chinese meal was peanuts and Jennifer concluded she had become allergic to peanuts. This frightened her because she knew that some people can get life-threatening reactions if they have a strong allergy to peanuts. So she went to an allergy centre to find out what was happening.

Allergy testing showed Jennifer had strong dust mite and grass pollen allergies. These were causing her sinus problems but certainly not her hives and facial swellings. None of the foods tested provoked a positive response. Conclusion: Jennifer's allergic reactions were not due to a food allergy. 'So what then,' asked Jennifer, 'could be causing this?' Fibre-optic inspection of her nasal cavity showed a grossly swollen nasal lining with fluid 'blistering' along the upper turbinates. Left unchecked, this would eventually trigger allergic nasal polyps. More importantly, the swelling was interfering with the delicate nerve ending carrying the sensations of taste and smell to Jennifer's brain.

It was explained that to get better she had to avoid specific E numbers (the chemical additives put in certain food products to colour, flavour and preserve them). She would also start a treatment plan to restore her nose and sinuses to normal and recover the lost senses of taste and smell. With full recovery she would enjoy good, wholesome food and not be so inclined to go for spice in her diet. Jennifer was also told that if she followed this plan she would improve very quickly. However, she was warned that, for reasons not fully understood, once withdrawn, the casual reintroduction of the banned additives could trigger very aggressive reactions. Dubbed 'heightened hypersensitivity', it's as if the body is taking a breather from all the junk thrown at it and warns that the next time one of the banned chemicals enters the system it will explode with allergic activity, producing hives, facial swelling, tongue swelling and even narrowing of the throat.

So what is the special diet for sinus patients who erupt in hives?

As I explained in Chapter 4, those with sinus problems (both adults and children) look for more tangy, spicier foods and flavourings. Unfortunately almost all tang and spice is artificially created using chemicals. These people can unwittingly make their condition worse (and add in an extra problem) by using artificially flavoured foods, especially in Indian and Chinese dishes.

As we also saw in Chapter 4, many chemical additives are used by the food and drink industry to colour, flavour or preserve food and drinks, such as crisps or fizzy drinks. Each additive is labelled by number, with the letter E attached; these are known as 'E numbers'.

So, as part of Jennifer's overall management she had to avoid the food additives listed in Chapter 4 (see page 36). Especially she had to look out for E621, monosodium glutamate. Jennifer was told to avoid poorly labelled products, or those bearing the phrases 'contains permitted additives' or 'contains permitted colourings and flavourings', or just saying 'colourings and flavourings'; she was also advised to avoid products coloured red, orange, yellow, blue, lemon or green, any of which might contain one of the listed agents, and to check tablets, capsules, lozenges and vitamin preparations, even the stripes in toothpaste. If she was unsure about the safety of any product, she was told not to buy it.

She stuck to these rules, and she did it. With her sinuses successfully treated, Jennifer improved dramatically. She's still sticking to the additive-free diet and remains well to this day. She still longs for the occasional Chinese takeaway.

There's no pleasing some people!

10

Summer sinusitis: hay fever and immunotherapy

Almost all sinus problems begin in the nose.

Aaaaccchhhhoooo! You just know it's that time of the year again. 'Get me a tissue quick.' Aaaaccchhhhoooo! 'For goodness sake pass the tissues.' Aaaaccchhhhoooo! 'I wish it would rain. I hate this weather.' It's the sneezing epidemic from hay fever. Perhaps the winter wasn't especially harsh and spring did drag on longer than usual, but suddenly summer arrives and there's a bounce to everyone's step. The days are longer, the nights shorter, the sunshine warm to the face. Newspapers carry features on gardening and the sound of lawnmowers almost drowns the background drone of traffic. These are wonderful, relaxing conditions for most people, but miserable for those with hay fever. While the rest of us haul out the barbecue and prepare for lazy outdoor evenings, a significant number dread putting their noses past the rear window. The cause relates to pollen sensitivity and affects about 20 per cent of the population, especially teenagers and young people. However it can erupt at any age. The symptoms include:

- sneezing
- blocked and runny nose
- sinus congestion with headaches, especially along the forehead
- itchy eyes
- coughing and occasional wheezing
- an itch along the roof of the mouth and the back of the throat
- a feeling of intense lethargy

Hay fever is an exquisite allergy to grass pollen (mainly) and mould spores. It is a particularly seasonal (especially mid-summer) problem but can drag on into early autumn. Allowing for weather variations, the pollen season starts earlier in the south of Europe than the north. In the UK and Ireland the aggressive sneezes can be heard first along the warmer western coasts. By the end of May high pollen counts can be detected countrywide (the pollen count measures the amount of pollen in the air over 24 hours). High levels of pollen occur on warm, dry and sunny days; low levels occur on wet, damp and cold days. Rain washes pollen out of the air. Pollen is released in the morning and carried higher into the air by midday. It descends again to 'nose level' in the late afternoon. Cities and dense urban areas stay warmer longer and hold pollen. Combine this with atmospheric pollution from car fumes and you can understand why city dwellers suffer more aggressive hay fever than their country cousins.

There is a group of people with allergy who have an all-year-round sinusitis that becomes dramatically worse in the summer. They usually have an additional dust mite or animal hair sensitivity which keeps the nose and sinus tissue constantly inflamed. Along comes a warm, sunny day with high levels of pollen in the air and suddenly their nose and sinuses become totally obstructed. They feel miserable, tired and exhausted. They have sinus congestion, itchy and red eyes and often wheezy chests. Old patches of healed eczema become irritable again and the urge to scratch becomes too much. What was once healthy skin now becomes dry, red and inflamed.

Avoiding pollen and reducing its effects

There are a number of things you can do to reduce your exposure to pollen, and to lessen the effects of an allergy to pollen. You many find some of the following helpful:

- Avoid areas of lush grassland.
- Keep house and car windows closed during the peak pollen hours of late morning and late afternoon.
- Wear wrap-around sunglasses to reduce the effect of the pollen grains on the eyes.
- If you can, avoid being outdoors in the late morning and late afternoon.
- Don't smoke, and keep away from smokers (passive smoking aggravates all allergies).
- Get someone else to mow the lawn.
- Choose seaside breaks for holidays, as offshore breezes blow pollen away.
- Check TV, radio and newspapers for the next day's pollen count and plan your schedule accordingly.
- Put a smear of Vaseline inside each nostril to ease the soreness and to capture pollen entering the nasal passages.
- Never sleep with the bedroom window open.
- Don't drive with the window open.

Remember to think about the foods you eat. There is a link, called the 'oral-allergy syndrome', where certain foods cross-react with specific environmental pollens and moulds. This triggers itching and slight swelling of the lips, tongue and the back of the throat.

For example, if you're allergic to birch pollen you may also react to celery, curry spices, raw tomato, raw carrot, apples, pears and kiwi fruit. If you're allergic to grass pollen you may also react to oats, rye, wheat, kiwi fruit and raw tomato. If your allergy is to weed pollen you may also react to raw carrots and curry spices. Mould allergy can sometimes cause reactions with certain yeast products.

What treatments can I take?

At the risk of annoying you, remember the golden rule of sinusitis management: *almost all sinus problems begin in the nose.*

For immediate relief an antihistamine is helpful in 'mopping-up' excess circulating histamine, the main cause of hay-fever symptoms. When buying an across-the-counter antihistamine, choose one of the newer 'won't make me drowsy' products (some older drugs control hay fever by forcing the patient asleep for most of the summer!). The antihistamine is often combined with a steroid nasal spray and special anti-allergy eye drops.

However, successful management depends totally on reversing the nasal blockage. Neither an antihistamine nor a steroid nose spray will unblock very congested nostrils. A short course of decongestants such as Otrivine (chemical name xylometazoline) may be needed to provide immediate relief and allow the usual medication to become effective. My preferred therapy is to use Betnesol nose drops in the 'head-back' position, as explained in Chapter 3 (see Figure 3.2). This strategy slowly restores the swollen nose and sinus lining to normal. It also relives the itching and irritability, and dries up the clear mucus flow associated with hay fever. Once the nasal cavity is unblocked the standard, very safe and effective nose sprays can then reach all areas under threat of further pollen challenge.

Here's a typical regime for an adult.

Betnesol nose drops for hay fever

- Get into the position suggested (see Chapter 3 for explanation).
- Instil two drops of Betnesol into each nostril.
- Stay in the position for three minutes.
- After the three minutes pinch the soft part of nose closed. Now lift your head to the normal position (some drops may spill out at this point but that's not important).
- Do this twice daily (preferably morning and evening) for seven days.
- On day eight start the nasal spray (Nasacort or Flixonase or

Avamys or Nasonex). The dosage is one squiff up into each nostril twice daily.

• An ongoing strategy until the end of the pollen season might be a nasal spray, one squiff into each nostril twice daily, combined with a non-drowsy antihistamine such as Xyzal (levocetrizine), Neoclarityn (desloratidine) or Zirtek (cetrizine).

In addition to the above treatments and strategies, there's now a more permanent way of dealing with allergy: immunotherapy.

Immunotherapy

Allergy management involves avoidance of what you are allergic to combined with treating the symptoms. For example, in sinusitis due to dust mite sensitivity special mattress covers and low allergy pillows are advised, while the snorting and sneezing is suppressed with medication. However, while such manoeuvres and treatments are indeed very effective, they do not alter your allergic status. In other words you are still allergic to dust mites and still get into trouble if the avoidance measures and treatments are relaxed or stopped. For almost all people with allergy this means many years (even a lifetime) of taking anti-allergy remedies.

Now a new therapy (or rather an old therapy updated) offers the chance to significantly reduce your 'allergicness' and maybe even to completely stop reactions. Immunotherapy entails taking exactly what you are allergic to, but in a modified form. At present the most convenient product, called sublingual immunotherapy, is a dissolvable tablet placed under the tongue and held there for two minutes. In North America and some European countries, immunotherapy is given by weekly injections. It's exactly the same principle, just a different mode of delivery. However, this is not very patient friendly. Taking time out to go to the same doctor, week after week, for a single injection is more than most people with sinus problems are prepared to do. The under-the-tongue version is more acceptable as a long-term course of treatment.

In medical jargon, allergen immunotherapy blocks the allergic reaction well upstream of the inflammatory response and may even prevent nose and sinus allergy (sinusitis) deteriorating to lung allergy (asthma). Moreover, its beneficial effect persists long after the end of the course of therapy.

Allergen immunotherapy is especially helpful with hay fever-induced nose and sinus problems. To summarize then, allergen immunotherapy:

- reduces symptoms significantly;
- reduces the amount of medication needed for comfort and relief;
- reduces nose and chest sensitivity to allergen irritation;
- reduces the risk of developing other allergies.

Why recommend immunotherapy?

Because it's the only therapy that offers the chance significantly to reduce or even stop anti-allergy medicines. More often than not, anti-allergy treatments are used daily for years, even for a lifetime. Anything safe and effective that might ease that considerable pharmaceutical burden is worth considering. The commitment to treatment is vital and this is important to understand, as you will be embarking on a minimum of three and possibly five years of therapy.

There is one product licensed in Britain and Ireland for grass pollen allergy sublingual immunotherapy. It's called Grazax (see <www.grazax.com>) and it's a dissolvable tablet that is placed under the tongue. It should be started well in advance of the pollen season to achieve the immune stimulation needed to try and induce a 'cure' of the pollen allergy. Grazax is taken daily for 52 weeks of the year for a minimum of three years. Highly allergic individuals may require a five-year course for final 'cure'.

Safety

The products used in sublingual immunotherapy have been thoroughly tested. Over 12 years, nearly one million treatments – corresponding to a total of 500 million doses – have been administered. Most side-effects were minor and of little significance (usually itching in the mouth, swelling of the lips or abdominal cramps). Rarely, cough, nasal irritation or asthma may be exacerbated. If there is a significant degree of swelling within the mouth, or even the faintest hint of throat swelling, then the treatment must be stopped and not restarted in case it provokes more serious responses.

At what age is it safe to use immunotherapy?

Immunotherapy is licensed for use in children aged five years and over for one product only (Staloral, made by Stallergenes in France: <www.stallergenes.com>). Grazax, mentioned above, is licensed only for those aged 5 years and above. At present this is for grass pollen-only nose and sinus problems but the company is working on a similar compound for those with dust mite allergy.

My own feeling (based on past experience in using injection immunotherapy) is that the benefits are best seen in young people. People 30 to 40 years old may achieve results, while for those over 50 years of age such therapy is probably not going to offer any extra benefit compared to standard anti-allergy medicines.

Long-acting steroid injections for hay fever

There is another product occasionally used for pollen sinusitis. Kenalog (chemical name triamcinolone) is a long-acting steroid (cortisone) injection. It comes as a single ampoule shot and lasts approximately six weeks at its 40 milligrams strength.

Most specialists in allergy and ear, nose and throat disorders avoid Kenalog because of potential side-effects. The drug is a steroid and consequently has the potential for a number of problems including suppression of natural cortisone production, dimpling of the skin and fatty tissue underneath the injection site, thinning of bones and wasting of muscle and tendons. So why even consider it?

Well, there is a small sub-group of severe hay fever sinusitis patients for whom standard treatments don't work. This includes people with significant mental or physical disabilities who cannot manage the daily ritual of anti-hay fever therapies. Also, long-distance lorry drivers and machine workers must be alert all the time. If the grogginess of hay fever combined with side effects of antihistamines impairs their concentration, a serious accident might happen.

A single and once-a-season, once-a-year injection of Kenalog will not cause side-effects. Indeed it offers this selected group of hay fever patients a decent quality of life during a time of year when we all like to be outdoors. It should not, however, be used more than once in the season.

11

Allergy testing

OK, your doctor has inspected your nose and sinuses, maybe checked your blood and ordered a CT scan for more information. She's decided that your sinus problem is almost certainly due to an allergy and she wants to know exactly what you're allergic to (and so do you). So she orders an allergy test. I do not want to confuse you with science or medical jargon but let's explore the basics of allergy.

What is allergy?

An allergy occurs when the body's immune system over-reacts to normally harmless substances (called allergens). These substances may be in the air or what you touch or eat. So the term allergen means anything that triggers an allergic reaction.

If you are an allergic person, and you come into contact with an allergen, your immune system produces a special kind of antibody (called IgE). Other cells release chemicals such as histamine that cause the symptoms you experience (blocked nose, itchy eyes, sneezing, wheezing, scratching, etc.).

Common allergens

Because this book deals with sinus-related health problems I'm only going to focus on the two types of allergens that cause sinusitis: environmental allergens (especially airborne ones, e.g. grass pollen) and ingested allergens (in other words, those we eat or drink).

The main environmental allergen is the dust mite – or, to be more precise, its faeces. Pollen, particularly from grass, trees and weeds, is another common allergen, as is animal dander (skin scales or flakes from the fur or feathers of animals). Mould and fungal spores are also common causes of nose and sinus problems and they too are carried in the wind.

Food allergy as a cause of sinusitis is rare. The commonest trigger is dairy products and often this is only convincingly proven by staying off all dairy products for a minimum of three months to see if your symptoms improve. If you do feel dramatically better, the diet is broken and any deterioration recorded. If it looks a dead certainty that dairy has caused your sinusitis, there is no treatment other than a dairy-free diet. However this should be planned in conjunction with a trained dietician. Dairy-free diets can cause nutritional deficiencies, especially in children. You don't want to create a new problem while attempting to solve an existing one.

Cigarette smoke is often considered an allergen but it is actually an irritant. This means it does not cause an allergic reaction; rather it makes the existing allergy worse.

Allergy symptoms

These depend on which part of the body is affected. For example, hay fever affects the eyes and nose, causing sneezing, a runny nose, watery and itchy eyes, irritated and itchy throat and a stuffy, blocked nose.

Eczema (also called dermatitis) is an allergic affliction of the skin causing itchy, red rashes.

Asthma is an allergic challenge to the respiratory system causing wheezing, breathlessness, chest tightness and a cough.

Allergies to foods, bites or stings can cause hives (doctors prefer the term urticaria because it's a strange term and using out of the ordinary words makes us feel important).

Diagnosing allergy

There are three types of allergy test:

- *Radioallergosorbent testing (RAST)*. This identifies exactly what you are allergic to through a blood sample. There are practical difficulties with RAST testing: it is expensive, the results take weeks to return and there is a limit to the number of substances that can be tested.
- *Serum IgE*. Another blood test which checks the number of allergy cells circulating in your body. This tells how allergic you are but *not* what you're allergic to.
- *Skin-prick allergy testing*. This is the commonest procedure used in sinus clinics. It is explained in detail below.

Skin-prick allergy testing

The surface of the skin is rich in mast cells. Mast cells hold the body's memory for allergy, in other words the cells recognize what you are allergic to.

There are also mast cells on the surface of your eyes, nose and sinuses, your mouth and tongue, throughout your breathing and eating tracts. They also run along the surface of the gut. In allergic reactions the mast cells 'explode', releasing a number of chemicals that cause problems. Where the reaction is localized (e.g. confined to the nose, sinuses and eyes in pollen hay fever) the problems stay localized (itchy eyes, sneezing, blocked nose, sinus congestion). Where the reaction is widespread (e.g. exposure to shellfish in a highly allergic person) the mast cell eruption can be so aggressive that it causes a total body response, which can occasionally be fatal.

With a skin-prick allergy test the doctor places a concentrated drop of allergy extract on to the forearm. Each drop contains an individual test substance such as dust mite, cat hair, horsehair, grass pollen and foods. Not every food is available in test form and occasionally fresh food will be used.

The test drop is brought into direct contact with the skin mast cells by pricking the surface with a sterile needle point and allowing the fluid to seep to a lower level. If you are allergic to a specific substance the mast cells underneath will 'explode' and a reaction (called a 'wheal and flare') appears. Simply put, the wheal is a red, itchy blister that forms over the test extract, and the flare is the associated redness of the skin.

The size of the central blister plus any surrounding skin redness tells the doctor what you are allergic to and how strongly allergic you are. Small reactions are not as important as large swellings. Large and very irregular reactions suggest high allergy. Large and very irregular reactions to food extracts suggest the possibility of a very aggressive and total body allergic response if that food is consumed. You can see colour photographs of skin-prick test reactions on <www.allergy-ireland.ie>, 'Your allergy consultation explained'.

The reactions you show on testing will be considered alongside the other symptoms you have and what the doctor discovers when she examines you before a final interpretation of the test is made.

Allergy testing: questions and answers

Why is allergy testing important?
Finding out what you are allergic to is an important first step to effective allergy treatment. When combined with a detailed medical history, allergy testing can identify the specific allergen(s) that triggers your sinusitis.

Who can be tested for allergies?
Adults and children of any age can be tested for allergies.

How long does it take to get skin test results?
Skin testing is fast and positive reactions usually appear within 20 minutes. Sometimes redness and swelling can occur several

hours after skin testing. The delayed reaction usually disappears in 24 to 48 hours, but should be reported to the allergy doctor or nurse.

Is skin testing painful?
Skin tests cause little or no pain. However, positive reactions cause annoying, itching red bumps which look and feel like mosquito bites. The itching and bumps are usually gone within 30 minutes.

Do any medicines interfere with allergy skin tests?
Yes: antihistamines and specific antidepressants block the 'wheal and flare' response of skin-prick tests. Before attending for an allergy test you must not be taking tablets or liquid of antihistamine medicines (please note, these are put into many cough mixture bottles). Antihistamine and steroid creams are also potentially troublesome for the same reason. Ideally you should not be taking steroid tablets, but this is not vital and will not significantly interfere with the result. If you have any doubt about medications, please check with your treating allergist.

When are allergy blood tests used?
Blood tests for allergy are used if you are taking a medicine that interferes with skin testing and cannot stop taking it; if you suffer from a skin condition so severe that there is no normal skin on which to perform the test; or if testing with a strong allergen might cause an especially unpleasant positive reaction.

How long does it take to get blood test results?
Because the blood sample must be sent to a laboratory for testing, it takes many days, even weeks, to get results.

How are skin-prick tests interpreted?
Skin-prick tests help find allergies to pollen, moulds, dust mites, animal dander, insect stings and foods.

A positive result is measured in millimetres of central wheal and outer flare (flare here meaning the redness of the skin).

There are positive (histamine) and negative (saline) controls to compare against and thus ensure accuracy of result.

With foods, a wheal of 6 mm and greater suggests that particular food will trigger an allergic reaction. The greater the size of the wheal, the more likely that the reaction will be aggressive.

With environmental allergens (such as dust mite, pollens and animal hair) the size of the wheal and flare is important but does not always reflect the symptoms. For example, a person will occasionally show a very large wheal and flare (say to dust mites) but not show many symptoms. Equally, a relatively small reaction (say to cat hair) in someone only recently exposed to cats is usually very important, as within a year of continuous exposure the allergic reaction will probably have increased significantly (as will the person's symptoms).

It's easy to perform an allergy test; the skill lies in interpreting the result and linking it to the person's symptoms.

The bottom line on allergy testing in evaluating sinusitis is this: the result must be interpreted in combination with your symptoms (your sense of unwellness), what the doctor finds when she examines your nose and sinuses and the outcome of any other tests. When she has the whole package she can then conclude with some certainty that your positive skin allergy test truly reflects the cause of your sinusitis. That decided, she will then offer appropriate anti-allergy advice. The more experienced the doctor, the wiser the advice you'll be offered.

Anti-allergy advice

If something significant shows on testing, you are likely to be offered one of three types of advice on controlling your allergy:

- Environmental control (based on results that suggest your sinusitis is caused by airborne allergens such as dust mites, animal hair, pollen grains, etc.).

- Dietary advice (based on results that suggest some food is causing your sinusitis. However this is quite a rare finding. Diets *are* recommended in certain types of sinusitis, as explained in Chapter 13).
- Immunotherapy.

Immunotherapy

As explained in more detail in Chapter 10 (see page 80), immunotherapy today offers a significant chance to reduce your 'allergicness' and maybe even completely stop reactions. It blocks the allergic reaction, and may prevent symptoms developing in the long term as well as in the short term. Allergen immunotherapy is especially helpful with seasonal pollen sinusitis, as well as all year round nose/sinus, eye and chest allergy due to a dust mite and pollen combination. Animal hair allergy may also be dealt with in this way, but I still feel it's wiser to avoid the animal. With problematic sinusitis, immunotherapy is the best choice for long-term management. However you will be taking medication while you undergo immunotherapy. This will gradually be reduced as the immunotherapy starts to become effective.

To recap, allergen immunotherapy:

- reduces symptoms significantly;
- reduces the amount of medication needed for comfort and relief;
- reduces nose and chest sensitivity to allergen irritation;
- reduces the risk of developing other allergies (especially important in young children with, say, a dust mite allergy, where there is concern that pollen allergy may also develop in time).

Changing your environment

As well as diet and/or immunotherapy, anti-allergy manoeuvres for chronic and debilitating allergic sinusitis include environmental changes. Dust mites, pollens, moulds and pet hair are the most important cause of sinusitis. Because they may not always be easily avoided, try minimizing the 'allergy load' in your home as described below. See also the pollen-allergy avoidance strategies listed in Chapter 10 (page 78).

Environmental control of dust mite and animal hair allergy

Dust mites live comfortably in mattresses, pillows, duvets, blankets, carpets, soft furnishings, curtains and similar fabrics. The female mites lay up to 50 eggs, with a new generation produced every three weeks. Each mite produces about 20 waste particles every day. When working on anti-dust mite regimes, concentrate on the bedroom:

- If your bedding (mattress, pillows, eiderdowns, bolsters) contains wool, kapok, cotton, horsehair, feathers or down with synthetic materials, change to polyester or dacron.
- Buy blankets and curtains made of synthetic fibres.
- Get rid of down, winceyette and flannel materials.
- Get rid of carpets and rugs. Here there really should be no compromise. Mites also thrive in carpeting, no matter how tight the pile. The floors of those with mite allergy should be wooden (no unsealed cracks), linoleum, cork-tiled or parquet. These surfaces are so much easier to clean and run a wet mop over.
- Get rid of cushions not filled with synthetic materials, as well as anything made from wool or cotton.
- Minimize dust collectors such as heavy drapes, bookshelves, tapestries, etc.
- Paint rather than wallpaper the walls of the bedroom.
- Get rid of teddy bears and other soft toys. Special 'life-is-not-worth-living-without' soft toys should be washed at least once a week and each morning put into the deep freeze for about three hours to kill off mites.
- Open the bedroom windows for at least three hours every day, even in very cold weather.

- Use a damp cloth when dusting. Anything else only redistributes the dust.
- Choose lightweight curtains that are quick and easy to wash at temperatures around 58 °C. Consider roller blinds.
- Remove fabric covered headboards.
- Use only a vacuum cleaner with a special dust filtration unit. Vacuum and damp dust at least once a week.
- A bed with a plain wooden or metal base is preferable to a divan.
- Where bunk beds are in use, the sinus patient should sleep in the top bunk.
- Do not allow pets into the bedroom.
- Do not smoke, or allow anyone else to smoke, in a sinus patient's presence or in any other room he or she is likely to use.
- Don't have the radiator on as much in the bedroom, perhaps just enough to take the chill out of the air. Mites love warm temperatures.
- All clothes, shoes, socks should be put away in drawers and not left lying around the room. No hooks on the back of doors allowing clothes to hang there.
- If possible, have built-in wardrobes rather than free-standing units.
- Mattresses, pillows and duvets should be aired regularly. If there is a spell of good weather, get the bedding outside and into the air and beat the mattress to clear excess dust.
- Encase the mattress, pillows and duvet with a special protective cover that is comfortable to lie on, but does not permit dust mites to penetrate through. There are a number of companies dealing with these products and the price difference between them is very significant.
- Choose your vacuum cleaner carefully. The best (and unfortunately the most expensive) are those with high dust filtration units. This means the collected dust is retained and not

Sedgley Library
Tel: 01384 812790

Borrowed Items 07/02/2019 12:43
XXXXXXXX0497

Item Title	Due Date
Miller's antiques marks	07/03/2019
Mensa IQ tests : a complete guide to IQ assessment	07/03/2019
Fighting fatigue : managing the symptoms of CFS	07/03/2019
Sinusitis	07/03/2019
How to trace your ancestors using a computer for the older generation	07/03/2019
Charles Dickens : a life	07/03/2019
Report on the sanitary condition of lower sedgley urban sanitarydistrict : 1	07/03/2019
Switch on your brain	07/03/2019
Overcoming anger and irritability : a self-help guide using cognitive behavi	07/03/2019
Sedgley and district	07/03/2019

Indicates items borrowed today

Thank you for using Sedgley Library
http://capitadiscovery.co.uk/dudley

recirculated. Look for models produced by Medivac, Electrolux, Miele and Dyson. Make sure the supplier hasn't removed the special filtration bag (it does happen).

- When you are vacuuming and damp dusting, try and do a thorough job at least once a week and remember to go under the bed with the vacuum cleaner.

NB: if you are a sinus patient and smoke cigarettes, don't waste time, money and effort on anti-allergy manoeuvres. If you continue to smoke you undo the good that the above measures might achieve. *Even more important*: if your child is troubled with his or her nose and sinuses and you, your husband/wife/granny/uncle/babyminder or whoever, smokes such that your child passively inhales then, again, don't bother with anti-allergy programmes. Cigarette smoking makes all allergy problems worse.

An excellent website to check is <www.healthhouse.org>. This is a US site developed by the American Lung Foundation and lists anti-allergy regimes in great detail. Some of the suggestions do seem a bit over the top but most are common sense and practical.

12

Don't blow your nose: nasal douching

Almost all sinus problems begin inside the nose.

Blowing your nose to relieve stuffiness may be second nature, but some specialists in ear, nose and throat disorders argue it reverses the flow of mucus into the sinuses. It also slows the natural drainage of the sinuses. Not what you'd expect to learn, I accept, but closer examination shows it to be true.

To test the concept, infectious disease investigators at the University of Virginia in the USA conducted CT scans and other measurements as subjects coughed, sneezed and blew their noses. In some cases, the subjects had an opaque dye dripped into their rear nasal cavities.

Coughing and sneezing generated little if any pressure in the nasal cavities. But nose blowing generated enormous pressure – 'equivalent to a person's blood pressure reading,' one researcher said – and propelled mucus into the sinuses every time. The same doctor said it was unclear whether this was harmful, but added that during sickness it could shoot viruses or bacteria into the sinuses, and possibly cause further infection.

According to experts in the Department of Ear, Nose and Throat at the New York University Langone Medical Centre, the correct method is to blow one nostril at a time and to take decongestants. This prevents a build-up of excess pressure.

In conclusion, blowing your nose can create a build-up of excess pressure in sinus cavities.

So what do you do if you're troubled with nose and sinus problems and experts warn against that most traditional of remedies for relief, blowing the nose? As your local policeman might say, 'keep your nose clean'. In medical jargon it's called nasal lavage – also known as nasal douching, nasal irrigation or sinus rinsing.

While some amount of mucus production from the nasal and sinus lining is normal, allergies and sinus infections can cause excessive mucus production. This excess mucus causes nasal and sinus symptoms such as a runny and stuffy nose or post-nasal drip. The key to symptom relief is to physically wash away this excess mucus and allergens, such as grass and tree pollen, dust particles, pollutants and bacteria from the nasal passages. This rinsing will reduce inflammation of the nasal membrane, allowing you to breathe more normally.

The principle of nasal douching

There are a number of benefits to nasal douching:

- It gets rid of any allergy-provoking material in your nose.
- It gets rid of any pockets of infection that might be forming.
- It clears your nose and makes it easier to breathe.
- It moisturizes your sinuses.
- It feels refreshing

All that is involved is squirting a solution of slightly salty water up your nose, letting it drip out, blowing your nose gently, then repeating. The mechanical action of flushing out thickened mucus cleanses the nasal passages, making it easier for the tiny hair-like cilia that line the nose to push the remaining mucus out.

There is strong support for nasal douching (irrigation, lavage, call it what you will) among the allergy and ear, nose and throat specialist communities. 'Many people who have sinus disease, allergies, or chronic infections are improved tremendously by lavaging their nose out once or twice a day,' says a top USA-based ENT specialist. 'And for those who have had surgery to open up narrowed sinuses, regular cleansing is a must. The main improvement they experience is the ability to wash out the cavity.'

'Even if antibacterial medications are added to the lavage solution, most of the benefit is from the mechanical rinsing of the nasal cavity,' says yet another ENT specialist at the Massachusetts Eye and Ear Infirmary. 'Among other things, the gunk you rinse out in mucus includes natural chemicals called cytokines, which promote inflammation. If you remove the mucus, you can actually reduce the inflammation. But people need to do it with salty water to wash out mucus.'

While large, controlled studies of nasal lavage for treating and preventing colds and sinus infections are hard to come by, the little data that does exist seems to support the practice.

One study of more than 200 people published in 2000 in the journal *Laryngoscope* found that after three to six weeks of nasal douching, subjects reported statistically fewer nasal symptoms. A 1997 study of 21 volunteers in the same journal found that lavage improved the speed with which nasal cilia were able to move mucus along. A 1998 study in children published in the *Journal of Allergy and Clinical Immunology* showed that lavage is 'tolerable, inexpensive, and effective'.

Nasal lavage devices

In Asian cultures nasal lavage has a long tradition. There it is considered a very effective and simple form of therapy with almost no side-effects and very low costs. The easiest way is to sniff the fluid from the palm of the hand. 'Nasal showers' are marketed in health food stores in the UK and this type of mechanical rinsing is claimed to free the nose of any congested secretions and mucus which create a breeding ground for bacteria.

The 'Neti pot' is a container designed to rinse the nasal cavity. In essence it is a device like a teapot with an angled spout that allows warm, salty solutions to be poured into the nose, one nostril at a time. Neti pot enthusiasts say that with regular use it is more effective for nasal allergy and sinus symptoms than over-the-counter medications. All Neti pots operate on the principle of gravity. Tilting your head and simultaneously raising the Neti pot allows the solution to flow through the nasal passages due to the effect of gravity. They are suitable for people who cannot tolerate even the smallest amount of pressure in the nasal passages.

Neti pots do have some disadvantages. Many Neti pots cannot hold enough solution for truly effective use – you may have to prepare the solution twice to get the large volume required, which is costlier and more time consuming – while most Neti pots do not allow the user control of the flow of saline solution into the nasal passages. But the biggest limitation is that gravity alone cannot create sufficient pressure to wash away all the undesirable nasal irritants. While it may provide immediate relief, long-term benefit is unlikely because most of the mucus, associated pollutants and bugs remain in place.

In the USA hydro pulse systems are popular. These units produce a gentle, pulsating stream to cleanse and moisturize the sinuses, remove foreign matter, crusts and other undesirable materials. There are a number of units available commercially and claims for effectiveness include 'massaging the cilia of the nose and sinuses to their normal, healthy state'.

Pulse sinus irrigation has been shown in clinical tests to make the nasal and sinus cilia – the body's first line of defence against foreign bodies entering the sinuses – move better after treatment, transporting mucus out of the sinuses faster.

Current medical literature indicates that large volume saline nasal irrigation, delivered with low positive pressure, provides superior symptom relief to people with sinus disease and nasal allergies. For an effective nasal rinse, you need to use a large volume (100–200 ml) of saline solution in each of the nasal passages, delivered with adequate positive pressure to displace the mucus, pollen and allergens from the passages.

Effective nasal irrigation devices must have the following:

1 the capacity to hold a large volume of saline solution (200–240 ml);
2 the ability to deliver the solution with low but adequate pressure into the nasal passages. The pressure must be sufficient that the saline can not only flow through the nasal passages, but also displace the mucus, pollen and allergens;
3 finally, the saline solution must travel up the nasal passage and out through the other nostril. Unless this entire flow cycle occurs, you may not achieve a thorough cleansing job. This fact alone makes nasal sprays unsuitable for true large volume saline nasal irrigation.

Large volume (240 ml) easy-squeeze bottle systems effectively satisfy the requirements for a true saline nasal irrigation. These allow the user to deliver the solution with sufficient pressure to thoroughly clean the nasal passages, while maintaining the head in an upright position (no tilting or twisting of the neck required). The user has complete control of the pressure and the volume of solution as it enters the nasal passages, allowing for a gentle and therapeutic experience. All mucus and associated dirt, etc., is displaced from the nasal passages, allowing the user to experience long-term relief when the product is used consistently.

I've looked at many commercially available products and experimented with those I could get hold of. And I've decided there is one product that stands out from the others: Neilmed Sinus Rinse.

This is essentially a plastic squeeze bottle that holds 240 ml of liquid. With it come small sachets that contain salt and baking soda granules in an isotonic combination ideal for nasal irrigation. To use, boil a kettle of water and let the water cool until it is just warm. Empty one sachet into the squeeze bottle and top up with the warm water to the level on the side. Make sure the granules are dissolved. At the top of the black cap on the bottle is an opening. This is held against one nostril opening (as per instructions below), with the head slightly tilted forward over a wash basin. Squeeze the bottle firmly: one half of the contents should go up one nostril and come down the other side. Pause, blow the nose gently and repeat the procedure on the opposite nostril. This washes the nose and sinuses clean, and clears away any debris, allergy material, bacteria, viruses, etc. that may be lurking on the nasal lining. It is cheap, easily carried and available in pharmacies countrywide. The salt and baking soda combination is remarkably refreshing for those with sinusitis and they are delighted by the non-medical components of the product.

Sinus irrigation is more or less the mainstay of treatment for people who have had sinus surgery, but it's something I recommend as a daily routine for anyone troubled with sinusitis (of whatever cause). In the USA, it's considered almost as important as brushing your teeth and combing your hair before going out for the day. Think of it as dental floss for the nose and sinuses.

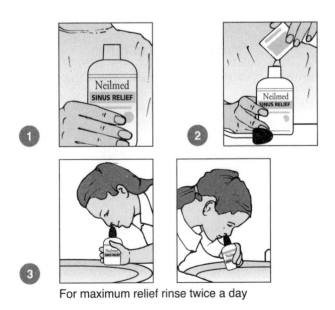

For maximum relief rinse twice a day

Figure 12.1 Sinus irrigation

13

Diets, self-help remedies and alternative therapies

While almost all sinus problems begin in the nose, factors well away from the nose can worsen sinus symptoms. In this chapter are some tips and advice along dietary/self-help lines to allow you to manage your sinus problems more effectively: not every therapy applies to every person with sinus problems, so check with your treating doctor before considering any. Knowing that many people prefer alternative therapies to traditional medicine, I've included management strategies from doctors who practice homeopathy and acupuncture. I can't guarantee they will help but you can be pretty sure they'll do no harm.

Sinusitis and acid reflux

If your sinusitis is caused by *acid reflux*, avoid the following:

- fried foods and those high in fat and caffeine
- chocolate
- tomatoes
- onions
- mint
- excessive alcohol

Cigarette smoke is a toxic substance that increases the production of stomach acid, possibly resulting in acid reflux. It is also a direct irritant of the nasal and sinus linings.

Sinusitis with diminished smell and taste

If you have sinusitis with diminished senses of smell and taste and you erupt in hives occasionally, then avoid foods that contain salicylate (see Chapter 4) and specific food additives (this is explained in greater detail in Chapters 4 and 9).

Salicylates occur naturally in certain foods, and depending on how troublesome your sinusitis is you may be told to avoid these totally, or, more likely, advised to consume them in small quantities only. Do not mix and match throughout this group such that you might unwittingly consume large quantities.

When taste becomes impaired in sinus problems the sensation of spice is the first to go. So, affected people – adults and children – tend to look for more tangy, spicier foods and flavourings. As I describe in Chapters 4 and 9, strong taste very often equates with chemical additives, identified by E numbers. Read the full explanation on pages 33–7, and particularly the list of food additives you should avoid as part of your overall management. Especially look out for E621, monosodium glutamate.

Take note also of the advice in Chapter 4 to watch out for poor labelling or the phrases 'contains permitted additives', 'contains permitted colourings and flavourings' or just 'colourings and flavourings'. Be careful of any product coloured red, orange, yellow, blue, lemon or green, and do check tablets and capsules, lozenges and vitamin preparations, as well as the stripes in toothpaste. Remember: if you are unsure about the safety of a product, avoid it.

Sinusitis and histamines

Some people with allergic conditions affecting the skin, chest and/or sinuses notice they feel worse after consuming certain foods or drinks. Occasionally this is due to high levels of *histamine* in the product. Most allergic individuals have excess histamine in their bloodstream (histamine is released during allergic reactions, which is why antihistamines are helpful). Eating or drinking histamine-rich products increases blood histamine levels and causes symptoms to flare.

The following foods and drinks contain high levels of histamine and should be avoided as part of your overall management of problematic sinusitis:

- Fish: tuna, sardine, anchovy, mackerel.
- Cheese: Emmental, Harzer, Gouda, Roquefort, Tilsit, Camembert, cheddar.
- Hard cured sausages including salami and dried ham.
- Vegetables: pickled cabbage, spinach, tomatoes and tomato ketchup.
- Alcohol: red wine (especially deep and heavy reds), white wine, sparkling wine, beer.

Sinusitis and asthma

If you have asthma and sinusitis, especially if complicated by nasal polyps, then the aspirin-free programme described in Chapter 4 (pages 33–7) is a 'must'.

Between 30 and 40 per cent (the statistics vary according to which expert you ask, but let's use these figures as a reasonable guide) of asthmatics with chronic (ongoing) sinusitis will become seriously allergic to aspirin/Disprin at some stage in their lives. This means that if they take an aspirin or Disprin they will get an aggressive flare-up of their nose, sinus and chest symptoms which occasionally can be life-threatening.

However, as I've already said, aspirin occurs in a wide range of across-the-counter medications, some complementary medicines, and even something as innocuous as teething gel. To recap what I've said in Chapter 4, the chemical name for aspirin is *sodium salicylate*. Salicylates occur naturally in certain foods: depending on your medical condition you may be told to avoid these totally, or, more likely, advised to consume them in small quantities only. See pages 34–5 for a list of these foods.

You may also need to avoid artificially flavoured foods and additives. Do please now turn to page 33 if you haven't already read this section, and carefully read the full story. It's quite detailed and you should make time to read it all through. A little care with what you eat is far better than an unpleasant – or even life-threatening – allergic reaction.

Alternative medicine, unusual and 'word-of-mouth' remedies

Chicken soup and lemon

Some researchers believe there are anti-inflammatory properties in chicken soup. So a 'soup and lemon juice' combination may help by reducing dehydration, mucus production and nasal congestion.

Vodka steam

Boil ½ pint of water and add a shot of vodka. Put the combination in a large bowl and cover your head with a towel and inhale the vapours. Maybe it's the soporific effect of the alcohol vapour that helps but some people, especially from Eastern Europe, swear by this remedy.

Vitamin C tablets in a cup of tea

The antioxidants in Vitamin C help modulate your immune reaction to viral head colds. And a cup of tea perks you up.

Chinese herbs

Yin Chiao herbs may have antioxidant properties that help with immune stimulation and speed up recovery from sinusitis. Antioxidants are widely used as ingredients in dietary supplements in the hope of maintaining health and preventing diseases such as cancer and coronary heart disease. Although some studies have suggested antioxidant supplements have health benefits, other large clinical trials did not detect any benefit.

Milk and garlic

Garlic is an antioxidant and anti-inflammatory agent, so it might help for those reasons alone. Milk hydrates.

Camomile steam baths

These are also worth trying, inhaled in a bowl with a cloth over the head. Other ethereal oils, for instance eucalyptus, pine tree, fir and peppermint, can be used to decrease swollen mucous membranes and dissolve secretion congestions. These ethereal oils should not be used when you are being treated with homeopathic remedies.

Homeopathy

According to my colleagues who practise homeopathy, when treating sinusitis the homeopath wants to know whether the sinusitis is of recent onset or long standing. If it's a persisting issue, then a full consultation with a reputable homeopathic practitioner is recommended. He or she will assess factors such as time of onset of discomfort, coincidental stress, lack of sleep, dietary changes, or exposure to the elements, to allergens, or to people who were possibly contagious. The sequence in which the symptoms developed may also be helpful.

Once the triggers to the illness are well defined, the actual symptoms and the way they affect the person assume more relevance. For example, the type and odour of nasal discharge, and the location and severity of pain, are important clues. Do you have a raised temperature? Fever suggests infection, but (at least in homeopathy) not always. The source of the infection is less important than the characteristic symptoms. As in most homeopathy there is no one specific medicine for sinusitis. Rather, your symptoms are matched with the properties of homeo-pathic medicines. The single best match is then given and the results assessed.

Pain described in small spots, rather than throughout the whole sinus zone, especially at the root of the nose, benefits from *Kali bichromicum*. Indeed this is the most frequently pre-scribed homeopathic medicine for sinusitis.

Mercurius solubilis is a close second in the list of homeopathic remedies for sinusitis. This would suit those with post-nasal drip, yellow to green nasal discharge, sweating with even slight exertion, bad breath and a metallic taste in the mouth.

Nux vomica or *Hepar sulphuricum* are used where the sinusitis is affecting the person's mood and making him or her ill-tempered. *Pulsatilla nigricans* is for even-tempered sinus patients. (Person-ally I don't meet too many even-tempered sinus patients!)

When a homeopathic medicine works for sinusitis, facial pres-sure and pain decreases, any fever eases and the nasal discharge becomes clear again. Overall the sense of sinus congestion lessens within 24 to 48 hours. Indeed the illness may simply go away at that point. Sometimes, even with best homeopathic practice, the sinusitis may progress into the chest, leading to a cough until the mucus is fully expelled.

Acupuncture

These are suggestions from my acupuncture doctor friend, who explains that long-term sinusitis is often caused by repeated infections by the common cold or influenza viruses. Part of the problem with this condition is anatomical. The openings into the nasal cavity are narrow and so if there is already inflam-mation, then further infection and inflammation makes the cavities prone to blockage. This results in stagnation of fluids in the nose and sinuses.

Within Chinese medicine, repeated invasions of common cold and influenza viruses occur because the *lung* energy is weakened. In addition, these infections interfere with the movement of lung energy, which in turn causes the fluids in the nose and sinuses to collect.

Diet can also play an important factor in the development of chronic sinusitis. Food items which are difficult to digest and are consumed on a regular basis will lead to the development and retention of *phlegm*, which will predispose one to sinusitis.

Acupuncture treatment for sinusitis is based on the symptoms you have when you visit the acupuncturist. When the symptoms are acute, treatment is aimed at clearing the phlegm from the nasal cavities and regulating the flow of lung energy. If the phlegm is yellow in colour then this indicates heat and points are selected to help the body clear this heat.

During symptom-free periods, or when the symptoms are mild, acupuncture treatment is aimed at strengthening the lung energy to prevent the invasion of pathogens (viruses). Other acupuncture points are selected according to imbalance in the body. It is also important to strengthen the digestive system and avoid food which is difficult to digest. This is because, according to a very important saying in Chinese medicine, phlegm is produced by the spleen and stored in the lungs. The *spleen* refers to the digestive system.

Chronic sinusitis can be difficult to treat. Sometimes it does not respond to acupuncture at all. The difficulty here relates to the phlegm being so thick and sticky that it is difficult to shift. There is also an underlying weakness in the body's energy which results in repeated invasions of viruses. To treat persisting sinusitis it is important to help the body eliminate the virus (phlegm), and to strengthen the body's lung energy (and spleen) to prevent future infections. Due to its stubborn nature, the best treatment for sinusitis is often a combination of acupuncture and herbal medicine. Treatment would be on a weekly basis initially.

Sinus massage

This is a quick and effective method to relieve your sinus pain. It also promotes drainage and relieves sinus pressure. However some areas of the face are very sensitive and too much pressure can worsen pain.

- Begin by gently massaging your forehead and cheeks, moving in small circles and working from the centre of your nose upwards.
- Find the V-shaped notch about 2 cm away from your nose, on the underside of your eyebrow ridge. Then, with both thumbs on either side, apply firm pressure here for ten seconds, release and repeat three times.
- Move your thumbs outward about 1 cm apart, and apply and release pressure here three times.
- With the pads of your middle fingers, feel for bony indentations at the bottom, outer edges of your nose. Apply and release pressure here also.
- With the fourth and middle fingers, apply upward and outward pressure at the top of your nose, between your eyebrows.
- With these same fingers, apply pressure along the underside of the cheekbone.
- Gently massage, in small circles, along your jawbone from your ear to your chin. Relax your face by yawning, then repeat.
- Gently massage or apply pressure to the top of your head, especially right around the crown. You can recognize the pressure points by noting the especially tender spots; that's an indication that some attention is needed at that spot.

Sinus massage can be a quick fix to restoring a normal lifestyle.

Herbal remedies

- *Liquorice root* helps reduce inflammation and stimulates the immune system to fight sinus infections. Be sure to take liquorice capsules that boost the immune system and not those for treating ulcers.
- *Eucalyptus* is a fragrant herb that soothes sore throats. It also has antiseptic properties and can help shrink swollen tissues such as sinus passages. It is available in convenient throat lozenges. You can also drink eucalyptus tea. Steep some eucalyptus in a large pot of boiling water and use as an inhalant to unblock nasal passages.
- *Peppermint* has anti-inflammatory properties and 'calms' swollen nasal and sinus membranes. You can get peppermint in tea or steep peppermint and breathe in the steam. Peppermint scent helps nasal breathing difficulties.
- *Ginger* has been known to relieve and prevent headaches. It is considered both an anti-inflammatory and analgesic. Buy in a reputable health food shop and take strictly according to instructions.
- *Lemon balm* is helpful in fighting off viruses and bacteria. Steep the dried leaves for ten minutes in hot water; strain and drink the tea warm. Alternatively, lemon balm tea can be used as a gargle.
- *Echinacea* boosts the immune system. There are claims that it kills respiratory viruses. Take in capsule form. Increase the dosage at the onset of illness and decrease after several days. *Do not take if you have an allergy to ragweed.*
- *Vitamin C and zinc* reduce the duration of colds as well as easing cold and flu symptoms. Since many sinus infections come from lingering colds the theory is that by starting vitamin C and zinc early you stave off infection. Take supplements in the form of capsules or lozenges during the winter months and at the onset of any sinus symptoms.

- Foods high in *antioxidants* help the immune system and prevent infections. These include blueberries, artichokes, red beans, cranberries and pomegranates. Add these to your diet to prevent sinus infections.

Note: Some herbal remedies can inter-react with prescription drugs, so check with your doctor or pharmacist before taking them.

Conclusion

As I've shown you in this book, persisting sinusitis can cause:

- allergic irritability in children
- asthma
- cognitive impairment in children
- cosmetic malformation of the facial bones in growing children
- decreased ability to concentrate
- decreased decision-making capacity
- exhaustion
- headaches
- hives (urticaria)
- impaired hand-eye coordination in children
- loss of senses of taste and smell
- migraine (as a trigger point)
- missed days at work or school
- nose polyps
- reduced physical activity
- school injuries
- sleep apnoea

And that's a lot of ill-health.

I've only had one sinus infection in my life (coming up to 60 years as I write) and I recall feeling like a bear with a sore head at the time. It's a discomfort I wouldn't wish on my worst enemy, let alone you, the reader. This book will help you understand why your (or your child's) sinuses are so troublesome and how you can start on the road to recovery.

Don't forget: *Almost all sinus problems begin inside the nose.* Keep your nose clean and your sinuses will stay healthy.

Index